Stroke, Body Image and Self-Representation

T0230864

Stroke, Body Image and Self-Representation provides a psychoanalytic reading of the subjective difficulties encountered by patients who have suffered a stroke. The book is based on the words of stroke patients and on their self-portraits, which are then compared with the words and portraits of subjects devoid of brain lesions. Pathological and normal self-portraits illustrate in very concrete terms the libidinal investment of our body parts.

The author's original data sheds an entirely new light on the subjective effects of a stroke. On the one hand, the permanent sequelae of a stroke can cause a narcissistic injury; on the other, a stroke may affect the brain circuitry involved in the patient's body image, undoing the normal narcissistic reactions. This may happen after right hemisphere lesions and cause spectacular symptoms, such as the personification of a paralysed hand or the apparent ignorance of a severe paralysis. This double aspect of a stroke is no small problem for rehabilitation therapists, who must avoid two pitfalls: considering any issue as psychological in nature, as if the brain lesion could not produce any organic changes, or, on the contrary, attributing any behavioural problems to brain dysfunction, as if the patient was devoid of normal psychological reactions. One of the aims of this book is to help therapists gaining their bearings in this little-known field.

In addition to this clinical interest, the author's psychoanalytic reading brings an original contribution to the physiopathology of cognition and self-representation. The data gathered by Catherine Morin show that self-representation cannot be considered only a cognitive operation. They also suggest that normal cognitive activity relies on both the stability of body image and the repression of the object. *Stroke, Body Image and Self-Representation* will appeal to psychoanalysts, psychologists, social workers, psychotherapists, psychiatrists, and rehabilitation therapists working with stroke survivors and patients with body image disorders.

Catherine Morin is a neurologist and a researcher (INSERM) with neurophysiological and psychoanalytic training. She has been involved in the rehabilitation process of stroke patients at the Rehabilitation department in the Hôpital Pitié-Salpetrière in Paris from 1972 to 2010. Since 1983, both her clinical and research work have been on body image and body schema disorders after a stroke. She is a member of Association Lacanienne Internationale and of the International Society of Neuropsychoanalysis.

Stroke, Body Image and Self-Representation

Psychoanalytic and Neurological Perspectives

Catherine Morin

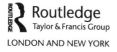
Routledge
Taylor & Francis Group

LONDON AND NEW YORK

First published 2018
by Routledge
2 Park Square, Milton Park, Abingdon, Oxon OX14 4RN

and by Routledge
711 Third Avenue, New York, NY 10017

Routledge is an imprint of the Taylor & Francis Group, an informa business

© 2018 Catherine Morin

The right of Catherine Morin to be identified as author of this work has been asserted by her in accordance with sections 77 and 78 of the Copyright, Designs and Patents Act 1988.

This book is a translation of a work previously published in French as *Schéma corporel, image du corps, image spéculaire: Neurologie et psychanalyse* by Éditions Érès, 2013.

Translation into English by Kristina Valendinova and Catherine Morin

Trademark notice: Product or corporate names may be trademarks or registered trademarks, and are used only for identification and explanation without intent to infringe.

British Library Cataloguing-in-Publication Data
A catalogue record for this book is available from the British Library

Library of Congress Cataloging-in-Publication Data
A catalog record for this book has been requested

ISBN: 978-1-138-93365-1 (hbk)
ISBN: 978-1-138-93366-8 (pbk)
ISBN: 978-1-315-62201-9 (ebk)

Typeset in Times New Roman
by Apex CoVantage, LLC

Contents

Foreword

It is difficult to imagine the experience of paralysis after stroke. To wake up after a sudden loss of consciousness, bedridden with little or no memory of how one got there, unable to feel or to move one side of the body, and therefore little able to move at all. To be returned to a state of utter dependence dominated by physical needs. To have no feeling from the paralysed side but, if the paralysed arm is placed across the body, to have the uncanny experience of one's own limb felt as a heavy immobile weight, sensed but not sensing, an object. *Mr E – Oh! All of a sudden – you are in good health, [. . .] you are normal, and then – snap! suddenly your life is . . . well . . . that's why . . . wrecks. Me, I say [we are] wrecks and I don't think I'm wrong . . .*

All this would be difficult enough without the additional, specific cognitive and psychological sequelae that accompany a stroke to the right hemisphere: hemispatial neglect, anosognosia and its variants, delusions of misidentification and reduplicative paramnesia. These are some of the most puzzling and bewildering effects of neurological insult. They have been the subject of myriad experimental cognitive investigations and elaborate theoretical formulations, the most important of which are clearly and cogently summarised in this book. But however ingenious, no cognitivist approach has been able adequately to account for these frankly bizarre phenomenologies, let alone for the subjective experience of these patients.

Some theorists working on the border between neurology/neuroscience and psychoanalysis have recognised a psychical dimension to these phenomena, and have interpreted the patients' utterances – in keeping with traditional object relations theory – as indicating repression with regression to primitive defences, denial, disavowal, splitting (for example, Solms and Kaplan-Solms in their "Clinical Studies in Neuro-Psychoanalysis" or

Feinberg's work on what he calls "neuropathologies of the self"). But such readings imply normal psychic architecture, as though the neurological insult the patients have suffered were simply a trauma, like any other, to be responded to and understood in a similar way. In fact, as Catherine Morin demonstrates so clearly, the profound disruption to spatial cognition and consequent disturbance to body image suffered by right-hemisphere patients produce a much more fundamental disruption to psychic architecture, to the sense of self, than is predicated by these accounts. This foundering of subjectivity on neurological shoals is the focus of this remarkable book.

Drawing on evidence garnered over nearly 30 years, this work is richly embedded in multiple disciplinary strands: neurology and rehabilitation medicine, cognitive neuroscience, and linguistics, as well as psychoanalysis. Morin adds a new dimension both to the cognitivist investigations of these patients and to conventional object-relations oriented psychoanalytic accounts, by drawing on a particular aspect of Lacanian psychoanalytic theory – Lacan's "mirror stage"– to ask what it is for a patient, a subject, to suffer these effects.

The patients' experience is analysed through both their utterances and their drawings. Speech was elicited in interviews about what they had been through, and remarked in the course of medical consultations or treatment sessions. Their language is analysed both linguistically – the use of pronouns, the position of the subject in relation to their speech – and psychoanalytically. Form and content are both revealing. The patients were also asked to draw themselves; the same care and attention is paid to 'reading' their self-portraits. The responses of patients with left hemisphere stroke or with paralysis but without brain injury are carefully reported, an essential backdrop to demonstrating the specificity of the right-hemisphere effects.

Incapable of understanding spatial relations, including the relations between their own body parts, and sometimes between their own body and those of others, the right-hemisphere patients seem not to occupy the same spatial dimension as their interlocutors. They do not initiate conversation but respond to questions as if from the recollected habits of daily life. They seem uninvolved in their own utterances, unengaged with those around them. Their pronominal world is altered, depersonalised: e.g. *One becomes a bit like a child again.* Their utterances seem to escape from an "isolated" psychic territory, a territory without spatial coordinates. The patients seem to inhabit a kind of Kleinian infant world of part objects, while the quality of their communication recalls Klein's description of schizoid patients in her "Notes on Some Schizoid Mechanisms": "their withdrawn, unemotional attitude. . . . [A] kind of detached hostility which pervades the whole relation to the (other). . . . The patient . . . feels estranged and far away, and this feeling corresponds to the . . . impression that considerable parts of the patient's personality and of his emotions are not available."

Their speech indicates an intricate interplay between body, cognition and psyche. It is not that an undamaged body, as such, is essential to the structure of the psyche; rather what is necessary is an intact body schema which relies on a representation of the body's intra – and extra – corporeal spatiality mediated through the specular image, which brings together the real body, its imaginary form, and its symbolic designation.

Seen through this lens of its fragmentation, it becomes clear that the mirror stage is not just a developmental moment to be passed through. Rather the specular image that it instantiates is constantly re-instated by lived experience, something of which we may only otherwise become aware in those transient moments in which we fail momentarily to recognise our own reflections. When the brain is damaged in such a way that the cognitive spatial representation of the body disintegrates, as it does in these right-hemisphere patients, so too does the psychic structure that constitutes a sense of self. What their utterances signify is not repression – as more conventional psychodynamic accounts imply – but precisely the opposite: what the patients give voice to is something that would normally be repressed but now is not.

What does it mean, in these circumstances, to say that the patients are unaware of their paralysis? Who have the patients become? What is 'the body' for them? Without spatial coordinates, to whom do the bodily 'bits and pieces' belong? One patient said of her paralysed side that it was a side "you cannot mourn because it does not exist"; one might equally suggest that there is no-one present any longer to do the mourning. The same patient said she sometimes had the feeling she had "forgotten her left arm at home", thus verbalising the idea that the arm remains outside the body image, 'left at home'. The fabric of conscious processing ruptured, questions are answered as if from a dream: . . . *"that's what I remember . . . I was lying next to this arm . . . I said that it was not my arm. I said that I was convinced that I fell asleep with my daughter in my arms. Thus, my daughter had put her arm around me. Thus it was her arm. Yes and I told everybody that it was not my arm since it was hers . . ."*

This marvellous book, now happily available to the English-speaking world, utterly transforms our thinking about these patients: in paying attention to the detail of what they say; in the inspired analysis of the patients' self-portraits; and in bringing Lacan's theory of the specular image to bear on these two sources of evidence, an entirely new way of thinking about the patients'experience is made possible.

Diana Caine, PhD
Consultant Neuropsychologist and Psychoanalyst
(National Hospital for Neurology & Neurosurgery, London)

Acknowledgements

My thanks go to Anne Salazar-Orvig and Diana Caine, who provided invaluable help for solving some tricky translation problems in the linguistic and neuropsychologic fields, to say nothing of their friendly support.

Copyright acknowledgements

Every effort has been made to contact the copyright holders for their permission to reprint selections of this book. The publishers would be grateful to hear from any copyright holder who is not here acknowledged and we will undertake to rectify any errors or omissions in future editions of this book.

Chapters 1 and 2 include excerpts previously published in: Morin, C., Thibierge, S. (2004). L'image du corps en neurologie: de la cénesthésie à l'image spéculaire. Apports cliniques et théoriques de la psychanalyse, *L'évolution Psychiatrique*, 69, 417–430. Copyright © 2004 published by Elsevier Masson SAS. All rights reserved. Reprinted by permission of the publisher.

Morin and Thibierge. (2006). Body image in neurology and psychoanalysis: History and new developments. *The Journal of Mind and Behavior*, *27*, 301–318. Reused by permission of *The Journal of Mind and Behavior* and the University of Maine.

Morin, C., Bensalah, Y. (1998). Self-portrait in adulthood and aging. *International Journal of Human Aging and Development*, *46*, 45–70. Reused by permission of the journal and SAGE Publications, Ltd.

Morin, C. (1995). La main en rééducation neurologique, réelle, symbolique, imaginaire? *Bulletin de l'Association Freudienne*, *62*, 15–19. Reused by permission of Association Lacanienne freud-lacan.com.

Chapters 4 and 5 include excerpts and a Figure from: Autoportraits de patients hémiplégiques. *La psychanalyse de l'enfant*, *14*, 1993, 140–147.

Excerpts from Condat, A., Morin, C. (2000). Hémiplegie, papotage et tripotage. *Bulletin de l'Association Freudienne Internationale*, *87*, 15–19. Both are reused by permission of Association Lacanienne freud-lacan.com.

Figures

Abbreviations

CVA   cerebrovascular accident
RHS   right-hemisphere syndrome
RBI   right brain injury

Introduction

In recent years, the representation of oneself and of one's own body as a coherent and stable unit has been the focus of numerous neuroscientific studies devoted to the questions of the self, self-consciousness or the first-person perspective. Very often, this research is based on the functional brain imagery of normal subjects performing a variety of mental tasks, which may consist of recognising a human or non-human body, or attributing certain gestures, mental characteristics, emotions and so on to oneself or others (see Legrand and Ruby, 2009). In these studies, the authors have felt entitled to break up self-consciousness into a number of components. However, this is a highly questionable postulate, since a crucial characteristic of self-consciousness is precisely that it cannot be defined as a simple sum of cognitive activities. Moreover, due to the experimental constraints of neuroimaging, the mental states examined are necessarily chosen from among those that can be produced 'on demand' during brief sequences. This is paradoxical, because the feeling of 'being oneself' greatly relies on the unconscious and permanent aspects of our psychic life. For example, as shown by the psychoanalytic experience, the operation of attributing a mental state to oneself is foiled by any ordinary slip of the tongue or parapraxis. The accompanying sense of embarrassment, the feeling that these phenomena are somehow alien to our normal discourse, is precisely due to their ability to reveal something intimate about our 'being ourselves'. Self-representation cannot therefore be treated as merely a question of cognitive functions (see Thibierge and Morin, 2010).

In the present work, I am not trying to find links between specific areas of the brain and cognitive or psychic activities, but instead examine the psychic effects of brain lesions from the perspective of physiopathology. Neurological semiology can in fact dissociate and highlight the diverse components whose combination permits us to see ourselves as unique and consistent individuals. Cerebrovascular accidents (CVAs) differ from both brain injuries and brain diseases, insofar as they can cause localised lesions and permanent alterations of the brain circuitry. The impact this may have on the psyche will depend on the specific areas of the brain that have been altered; the principal characteristics of this impact can regularly be observed in patients with the same localisation of the damage. Some of these psychic consequences may affect self-representation. The principal aim of this book is to describe these neurological disturbances of self-representation in psychoanalytic terms.

A CVA is caused by either a stoppage in the blood supply or bleeding in one or several brain areas. The patient may recover in only a few minutes, but his life can also suddenly change: someone who had previously considered himself 'healthy' can fall into the category of, first, a 'life-threatening emergency' and then 'disability'. Although much progress has been made in terms of CVA prevention and early management, it still remains one of the leading causes of death and disability (see Féry-Lemonnier, 2009; Feigin, Lawes, Bennett and Anderson, 2003; State of the Nation, 2017; National Center for Health Statistics, 2016). Because the brain is organised into specialised areas, a cardiovascular accident can cause a variety of deficiencies. These can affect not only the motor or perceptive functions (hemiplegia, i.e., paralysis of an arm, leg and/or face, balance disorders, sensory or visual disorders), but also the higher functions (language, spatial orientation, gesture programming) and behaviour. The resulting impairment and disability can thus be multifactorial and are specific to each stroke victim. However, regardless of its actual consequences, CVA is a stigmatising affliction. The mere notion of having suffered brain damage suggests that the patient's intellectual functions have become diminished. Stroke patients are suspected of having overindulged in the good things in life; they are enjoined that, from now on, they need to manage the risk factors in their lives (Morin, Salazar-Orvig and Piera-Andrès, 1993; Baumann and Aïach, 2009). If they are hemiplegic, their distorted posture and "crooked" mouth represent a deviation from the "proper" body image.

If, once the CVA has been diagnosed and treated, the patient is thought likely to suffer from disabling sequelae, he will be admitted to a rehabilitation unit. There, he will encounter numerous paradoxes and contradictions.

While he is still depressed and devastated by his altered self-image, he is forced to learn about the concrete consequences of his accident in great detail. His family is overjoyed that he has survived, he is congratulated on making good progress, but soon he discovers that the latter has its limits: he can move around, but he hobbles; he can move his leg, but not his arm. The patient also discovers that 're-training' often consists in learning how to cope with the lasting consequences of the accident. This development may not seem very different from that of any patient suddenly having to cope with a disability, but the fact that the injury originates in the brain makes the picture more complicated. On the one hand, the patient is affected by the stigma of a stroke (Goffman, 1963); on the other hand, some brain lesions do produce changes in the patient's psyche and affect cognition. Right hemispheric lesions, in particular, may disturb body representation. These disturbances create certain deficits (inability to recognise one side of the body as one's own, inability to perceive one side of the environment, being unaware of left-side hemiplegia); in addition, these deficits very often involve pseudo-delusional ideas regarding the ownership of the paralysed body and its various parts.

Rehabilitation medicine gives a neurologist access to certain aspects of the CVA that ordinarily escape our attention during more acute treatment. It offers a unique research opportunity for our understanding of the relationships between the physical body, body image and identity. The long period of hospitalisation (often many weeks or months) brings the patient into regular contact with a number of interlocutors (physicians, psychologists, students, physiotherapists, social workers, auxiliary workers, nurses, etc.), to whom he may communicate, in various forms, something about his body and his distress. At the same time, the great variety of patients admitted to a rehabilitation unit makes it possible to carry out comparative studies: some patients can have no brain lesions at all; those who have suffered a CVA may only have sensorimotor deficiencies, but they can also suffer from a body representation disturbance. Comparing these different types of patients is of theoretical interest, since it permits us to separate the individual components of what we call 'identity'. However, this research also has clinical implications. Every disabled patient is in fact at risk of being considered psychologically 'special'. His interlocutors may expect him to exhibit certain types of behaviour (Morvan and Paicheler, 1990) or be surprised if he expresses his emotions just like anybody else

(Zola, 1982). If the disability is due to a brain lesion, any words or behaviours that deviate, however slightly, from what therapists think of as 'normal' are likely to be attributed to the brain injury. This represents no small problem for rehabilitation therapists, who must avoid two pitfalls: considering any issue as psychological in nature, as if the brain lesion could not produce any organic changes, or, on the contrary, attributing any behavioural problems to a brain dysfunction, as if the patient had no right to or were devoid of normal psychological reactions.

One of the basic theoretical premises of this work is the psychoanalytic notion of the *specular image*, which has the advantage of weaving together the real physical body, its representation, self-image and subjectivity, thus avoiding the never-ending debate of mind–body duality or unity. The psychic consequences of a CVA can be described in the following terms: Every stroke causes a narcissistic injury; every 'rehabilitation' involves a process of mourning and depression. However, damage to the right hemisphere of the brain, which alters both the body schema and body image (Lhermitte, 1939/1998), may provoke a genuine disintegration of narcissism, where the normal imbrication of the body image and the object – in the psychoanalytic conception of the term – can suddenly come undone. This distinction is very important, since the current literature on the psychological effects of stroke, even when it describes these phenomena using the notions of 'self' or 'identity', generally seems to ignore the specificities of right-hemisphere lesions (see for example Ellis-Hill and Horn, 2000; Keppel and Crowe, 2000).

I will start by presenting the key notions regarding the body schema and body image, and discuss what is meant by identification in psychopathology. The patients' discourse and self-portraits will then be described and analysed in detail.

References

Baumann, M., Aïach, P. (2009). L' "aidant principal" face à l'AVC d'un proche. *Médecine*, *5*, 184–188.

Ellis-Hill, C.S., Horn, S. (2000). Change in identity and self-concept: A new theoretical approach to recovery following a stroke. *Clinical Rehabilitation*, *14*, 279–287.

Feigin, V.L., Lawes, C.M., Bennett, D.A., Anderson, C.S. (2003). Stroke epidemiology: A review of population-based studies of incidence, prevalence, and case-fatality in the late 20th century. *Lancet Neurology*, *2*, 43–53.

Fery-Lemonnier, E. (2009). *La prévention et la prise en charge des accidents vasculaires cérébraux en France. Rapport à Madame la ministre de la santé et des sports.* Retrieved on 26/6/2017 from http://www.ladocumentationfrancaise.fr/rapports-publics/094000505/index.shtm.

Goffman, E. (1963). *Stigma: Notes on the Management of Spoiled Identity.* Englewood Cliffs: Prentice-Hall.

Keppel, C., Crowe, S.F. (2000). Changes to body image and self-esteem following stroke in young adults. *Neuropsychological Rehabilitation, 10,* 15–31.

Legrand, D., Ruby, P. (2009). What is self-specific? Theoretical investigation and critical review of neuroimaging results. *Psychological Review, 116,* 252–282.

Lhermitte, J. (1998). *L'image de notre corps.* Paris: L'harmattan. (Originally published 1939)

Morin, C., Salazar-Orvig, A., Piera-Andrès, J.B. (1993). L'hémiplégie après accident vasculaire: ce qu'en disent les patients en rééducation. *Annales de Réadaptation et de Médecine Physique, 36,* 3–17.

Morvan, J.S., Paicheler, H. (1990). *Représentations et handicaps. Vers une clarification des concepts et des méthodes.* Paris: CTNERHI.

National Center for Health Statistics. (2016). *Cerebrovascular Disease or Stroke.* Retrieved on 20/2/2017 from www.cdc.gov/nchs/fastats/stroke.htm.

State of the Nation. (2017). *Stroke Statistics.* Retrieved on 20/2/2017 from www.stroke.org.uk/sites/default/files/state_of_the_nation_2017_final_1.pdf.

Thibierge, S., Morin, C. (2010). The self and the subject a psychoanalytical perspective. *Neuropsychoanalysis, 7,* 81–93.

Zola, I.K. (1982). Denial of emotional needs to people with handicaps. *Archives of Physical Medicine and Rehabilitation, 63,* 63–67.

Chapter 1

Body schema

A number of psychoanalysts have made a distinction between *body schema*, an anonymous neuronal organisation, and *body image*, which is subjectively invested by its owner (Berthaud and Gibello, 1970; Dolto, 1984). Other authors have contrasted the automatic functioning of the body schema with the "reflexive intentionality" directed to the body image (Gallagher, 2006). In any case, since Bonnier (1902) and Head (Head and Holmes, 1911), most researchers have agreed on the following postulate: Some brain circuitry structures a non-conscious body representation whose functioning we remain unaware of. This body schema allows us to automatically adjust our movements to the surrounding space (see Coslett, 1998). Such definition might lead us to place the body schema in the physiological realm rather than in the psychological, subjective field. However, it is in fact impossible to speak of the body in a 'neutral' way and this holds true for the body schema as well: We cannot talk about it without necessarily 'subjectivating' it. This becomes clear when looking at the history of the notion itself, which was introduced by Pierre Bonnier and Henry Head in the early 1900s (see Morin and Thibierge, 2004; Morin and Thibierge, 2006). Previously, the term that was used to refer to the body representation was *cenesthesia*, a notion that Bonnier argued should be abandoned in favour of his concept of body schema.

Cenesthesia

Cenesthesia (Hübner, 1794, quoted by Starobinski, 1977) was first defined as "a general sensitivity (*Gemeingefühl*), which represents the state of the body to the soul, while sensitivity informs it about the external world, and inner sense (*inner Sinn*) provides it with representations, judgments, ideas and concepts". Schiff (1894, quoted by Starobinski, 1977) later explained the function of cenesthesia:

> If, for example, an irradiation (from excitation toward centres) goes to a sensory centre, it will awake there the image of a colour, a tone or an object; an auditory impression may thus produce a visual sensation or an auditory impression or both together; such a secondary sensation will in turn produce a tertiary one and so on. In this way, a unique sensation may awake an infinite chain of central sensations, of sensory images, and, since all our thought moves in such images or, to express it more exactly, is nothing but a series of central images, i.e., of excitation of central end of sensory nerves, it happens that a sensation may produce a series of thoughts which, when linked to the primary sensations, must complete or rather create cenesthesia.
>
> (quoted by Starobinski, 1977, pp. 7–8, translated for this edition)

From this description, cenesthesia seems to be an essential element of human psychic life. In line with this, Séglas (1895) considered that disorders of cenesthesia were chiefly responsible for melancholia: according to him, "due to disorders that happen in the field of organic functions, the normal cenesthetic state of well-being produced by the harmonious consensus of organic sensations is replaced, once the balance has been disrupted, by a new and uncomfortable state of general unease"; this state is the "first cause of moral pain". Similarly, Dupré and Camus (1907) wrote:

> We propose to designate under the term of cenestopathy the distortions of those sensations that continuously reach the brain, coming from all areas of the body, and which in a normal state do not attract our attention through any particular characteristic in either their intensity or their mode. We know how important the field of cenesthesia is; beneath the field of conscious perceptions, it constitutes the primary foundations of our personality.
>
> (Dupré and Camus, 1907, p. 616, translated for this edition)

Psychic life is thus thought to consist of interactions between the body and the external world, both of which are at the origin of multiple stimulations, the combination of which constitutes the psyche.

The invention of body schema

When using the term *body schema*, one ordinarily refers to the "postural model of ourselves" proposed by Head and Holmes (1911). Head considered this model as a basis for representing one's own body: all new perceptions are referred to this "postural standard". Head insisted on its plasticity, on the fact that it is continually revised and updated. However, it was Pierre Bonnier (1902) who first introduced the term "schema"; this new term linked body representation to a form, rather than a set of more or less defined sensations. Bonnier believed that "the word cenesthesia cannot have any valuable signification in either physiology or psychology, since it does not involve the notion of topographic figuration, which is necessary for any definition of corporeality". Our "sense of attitudes", Bonnier claimed, "gives us an idea where each part of ourselves is located, and is the basis of any sense of orientation, be it objective or subjective and psychic. Its object is the topographic figuration (σχηεμα) of our ego. I have also suggested the term *schematia* for the kind of images created by this sense". It is worth noticing that the formula "topographic figuration of our ego" explicitly associates body representation to the psychic agency Bonnier calls the ego. He adds: "The topographic distribution of things around us, in relation to ourselves and to each other, which allows us to localise sensations outside, creates the notion of objectivity; in the same way, the notion of subjectivity depends on the localisation of things inside ourselves, and these two terms, of ego and non-ego, arise from the most direct operations of the sense of attitudes" (Bonnier, 1902, p. 147). As Bonnier and Head had argued, it has been confirmed that body schema mainly consists of spatial relationships and does not directly depend on sensory input. This was shown by a unique observation reported by Paillard (1999): His patient, who was deprived of any conscious sensitivity in one side of her body, was nevertheless able to precisely locate a tactile stimulus on this side, meaning that she retained a topographic representation of an insensitive bodily area. It should be noted that the term *body schema* is mostly used in reference to limbs, i.e., to the visible parts of the body that are involved in our gestures and movement in the outside world. The term is very rarely employed when speaking of anal, urethral or sexual areas or viscera; indeed, these body parts are absent from the canonical representation of the human body, as seen in drawings of school-age children or in the drawing made as part of the Harris-Goodenough test (Harris, 1963) or "Draw a Person" test (Machover, 1953).

The body schema is constantly updated; it is progressively built throughout childhood and integrates the modifications that accompany the process of ageing. However, it is also remarkably stable, since it resists the traumatic or artificial changes of the physical body (Lhermitte, 1939/1998). This stability is shown by the amputees' illusions (phantom limb): Despite the amputation of a limb, the body continues to be represented as a whole and perceptions are referred to this unaltered schema. Aristotle's illusion also shows that the body schema may prevail over sensory information. This illusion is obtained by placing one object (e.g., a pencil) between the external faces of two crossed adjoining fingers, i.e., between two areas that cannot but touch different objects in the physiological position of fingers. When the fingers are crossed, the subject then perceives two objects. In this case, the information brought by the cutaneous finger receptors is misinterpreted because of the topography of body schema. The illusion also exemplifies the relationship between space and body schema: from the 'brain's point of view', the spatial zones external to the two adjoining fingers are necessarily represented as separate spatial zones. Indeed, the brain's ways of processing the body and space are intertwined. This is why Lurçat and Wallon (1962) chose the title *Postural space and surrounding space (body schema)* [*Espace postural et espace environnant (le schéma corporel)*] for their paper on the development of spatial notions in children. They wrote: "Our research has shown that [. . .] the body schema was made up of various types of relationships between space, postural space and surrounding space, and that we could not study body schema without taking into account the position of the body in space and without defining the relationships between the body and the acts the children mimicked or performed with objects on other people's bodies" (p. 2, translated for this edition). This passage also implies a relationship between body schema and action.

Body schema and space

The relationship between body and space representation can be grasped by looking at what happens when it is artificially inverted. This inversion can be produced experimentally in normal subjects, by asking them to wear ocular prisms: This makes the subject perceive the right-side space on his left side and vice versa. Such experiments alter the representation of both body and space.

Scholl (1926), quoted by Schilder (1935/1999, p. 108), described how he felt after having worn ocular prisms for several days:

> In regard to the limbs and other parts of the body, the pre-experimental image intruded into the actual perception. Arms and legs which were actually seen were localized in a double way: There was the localization in which they were seen; but in the background there was the previous localization, closely related to muscle sensations and touch. [. . .] When one side of the body approached an object, the touch came from the opposite side to that expected.

Body schema, action, sense of agency

Space is where our gestures and movement take place. Following Merleau-Ponty (1945/2012), many authors have claimed that the body "carries along" its own space and this space only exists as the space where the individual may engage in action. It is therefore necessary that we mention the notion of the "sense of agency", i.e., the ability to acknowledge oneself as the author of one's gestures (see Jeannerod, 2003). One way of studying agency is showing subjects videos of hand and finger movements while they are simultaneously performing such movements themselves. The videos may either show the movements actually performed by the subjects or show other movements performed by the experimenter. Normal subjects are able to recognise their own movements, an ability which implies an organised body representation.

Body schema and body image in cognitive neuropsychology

In today's cognitivist research, the term *body image* is used to designate a body representation different from the body schema, but this difference has little to do with the distinction between schema and image underlined by psychoanalysis. When using this term, some cognitivist researchers think of the multiple verbal representations of the body, its different parts, its orientation in space and its spatial relationships with other bodies (Buxbaum and Coslett, 2001). Unlike body schema, these notions are acquired by learning (children are taught the names of body parts, the notion of left and right, etc.). Other authors also refer to the "visual body image", a term first introduced by Head, which, however, takes into account only the visual perception of one's body (Holmes and Spence, 2007). The "rubber hand illusions" illustrate this predominant role of visual perception: in this experimental framework (Botvinick and Cohen, 1998), normal subjects see a fake rubber hand instead of their own hand, which is hidden to them. When the experimenter stimulates the fake visible hand and the true hidden hand simultaneously, the subject 'feels' the stimulation in the fake hand, as if he had incorporated the rubber hand in his body schema.

Body schema and space representation acquisition

As shown by the progressive acquisition of equilibrium and motor skills in the course of a child's development, the process of constructing the body schema continues throughout childhood, but it is completely unconscious. As we know – but it is worthwhile to recall – spatial orientation is acquired in all daily life activities, for example when the child learns to dress himself, as well as through contacts with other people (teachers, school fellows, parents). The work of Liliane Lurçat (1974) has helped shed light on the stages involved in children's thinking about their peripersonal space, about the orientation of objects in this space and their mutual relationships. The errors made by children show that this acquisition initially follows a self-centred and anthropomorphic mode.

Both body schema and space orientation are thus constructed, each in its own way, throughout childhood. However, certain intriguing phenomena have raised the question of whether body schema might not develop on the basis of an innate, 'pre-wired' structure. These phenomena include, on the one hand, the occurrence of phantom limb illusions in individuals with phocomelia (who were born with upper limb abnormalities) and, on the other hand, the early motor imitations performed by newborns (Zazzo, 1988). These imitations indeed imply that infants have innate abilities, but not that these abilities refer to any kind of form or structure of the human body already embedded in the newborn's brain. Indeed, the relationships between children, their fellows and the adults they meet involve a variety of imitation behaviours. Early infant imitation might be linked to the imbrication of motor and sensory representations (Nadel and Decety, 2002), which may be built before birth by the sucking activities of the foetus (Gallagher, Butterworth, Lew and Cole, 1998). Interactions between the representations of one's own body and other bodies (Nadel and Decety, 2002) might account for the occurrence of phantom limb phenomena in phocomelic individuals.

The representation of one's own body and the bodies of others

Brain representations of one's own body and other persons' bodies pertain to certain shared areas of the brain (Decety and Sommerville, 2003). The unconscious representation of one's own body would thus be indissociable from the representation of other bodies and their movements. We are all familiar with people who mimic the lip movements of the person they are listening to. The discovery of mirror neurons offers a scientific explanation of this everyday phenomenon. Mirror neurons have been found in monkeys. They are situated in the ventral premotor cortex and in the inferior parietal lobule; they are activated when an individual looks at another individual who is performing certain gestures (Rizzolatti et al., 2006; Preston and de Waal, 2002). Functional magnetic resonance imagery (fMRI) recordings in normal subjects and intra-cerebral recordings in epileptic patients suggest that a mirror neuronal system might exist in the human brain as well (see Mukamel, Ekstrom, Kaplan, Iacoboni and Fried, 2010). The 'crossed' representations of oneself and the other, the interactions between perception and movement, might thus be crucial to building the body schema.

Hence, we could consider that the notion of body schema refers to a set of abilities involved in our moving and handling activities. This set of skills is acquired non-consciously, in a relationship with others. This implies that neurological body schema disorders – visual hemineglect, apraxia or dyspraxia – necessarily involve certain subjective aspects, which go beyond the simple and understandable psychological reactions to neurological deficiency. They may also include specific effects linked to the disorganization of the body schema.

Body schema disorders

Hemineglect

Hemineglect (Heilman, Watson, and Valenstein, 2002; Vallar, 2015) means not taking into account the stimuli that come from one side of the body or the one half of the surrounding space that is opposite to the hemispheric brain lesion. Left hemineglect occurs following a right-hemisphere lesion in a right-handed patient; it is much more frequent and more disabling than right hemineglect. Left hemineglect has detrimental consequences in everyday life: Patients may omit their left side when dressing or shaving, while doing their hair or putting on make-up. Most often, body hemineglect is associated with space hemineglect. Figure 1.1 illustrates the concrete consequences of space hemineglect: while making cookies, the patient does not use the left half of the baking tray and piles up all the pastry shapes on the right.

A variety of clinical and experimental data have shown that hemineglect does not result from a perceptual disorder. On the one hand, patients who only suffer from lateralised sensory or visual disorders are aware of their deficiencies and try to make up for them. They do not forget to either shave or put on make-up on one side of their face, nor do they only eat food from the right side of the plate. On the other hand, left hemineglect does not concern only visual or sensory perceptions. Patients may also neglect noises or voices that come from their left side. In addition, hemineglect does not mean that the stimulus is in fact not registered in the brain. This is perfectly obvious in the cases of reading disorders induced by left hemineglect. When asked to read words aloud, patients with left hemineglect could not do so, because they omitted the first letters and only pronounced those on the right (Berti, Frassinetti and Umiltà, 1994). However, further tests showed that they had in fact correctly 'recorded' the meaning of the very words they could not read out. A variety of paper-and-pencil or computerised neuropsychological tests may be used for diagnosing and assessing hemineglect. Most of them consist in copying pictures or geometrical figures, or in spotting significant elements that have been dispersed among distractors (Figure 1.2).

Several psychophysiological mechanisms might account for hemineglect (see Kerkhoff, 2001). Some authors consider hemineglect as a difficulty

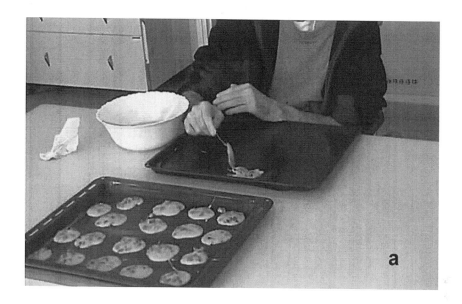

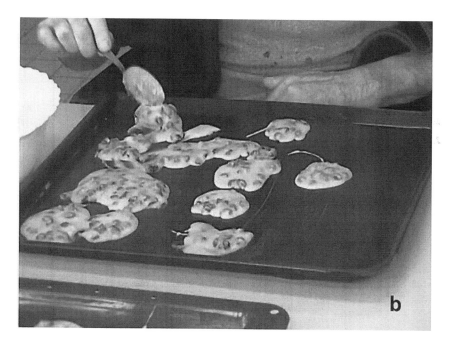

Figure 1.1 Left hemineglect in preparing shortbreads
The patient was asked to put the slices of pastry on a baking sheet as on the model sheet; (a) the patient puts the first slice in front of the model; (b) the final result: all slices but one are to the right of the sheet, most of them squeezed into the right-hand quarter.

Photographs taken by Hélène Migeot and Stéphane Vincent

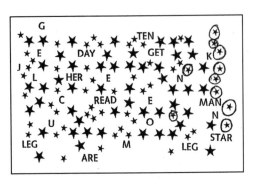

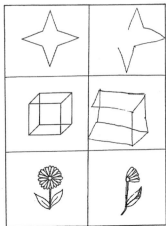

Figure 1.2 Left hemineglect in paper-and-pencil tests

(a) The patient (Mr E) was asked to circle all the stars in an 8.3 × 11.7 inch sheet (landscape orientation). The patient began on the right and circled only seven stars on the right edge of the sheet; (b) the omission of the left parts in copying pictures and geometrical shapes.

Source: Morin, Thibierge, Perrigot, Right brain damage, body image and language: A psychoanalytical perspective, *Journal of Mind Behavior*, 2001, 22, p. 76.

of acting in one hemispace, due to a lack of intention to move into the left space or explore it (see Bartolomeo, d'Erme, Perri and Gainotti, 1998). For others, hemineglect represents a disturbance of spatial representation: Bisiach (Bisiach and Luzzatti, 1978; Bisiach, Luzzatti and Perani, 1979) showed that patients with hemineglect have a hard time imagining one half of the space, whether it includes familiar places or abstract objects and shapes. For example, we asked a patient with left hemineglect which monuments she would see if she were standing in the Place de la Concorde in Paris and facing away from the Tuileries gardens. She then could only name one element on her left (the bridge), while she listed a whole series of buildings (the Hôtel de Crillon, rue de Rivoli, the Champs Elysées) that would be located on her right or directly in front of her. When asked to reverse her point of view (and imagine that she is now facing away from the Champs Elysées), she again only named one building on her left (the Hôtel de Crillon), but made the point of listing many of the buildings along the Seine on her right. Most of today's rehabilitation procedures are based on a third hypothesis, namely that patients with hemineglect suffer from a difficulty of allocating attention to the left side of their space, or of disengaging attention from the right side. Whichever the mechanism at stake, patients usually neglect both their left hemispace and their left hemibody; this confirms that there is indeed a close relationship between body and space representation, a relationship we also observe in patients with disorders of skilled movements (apraxias, dyspraxias), who too suffer from a disturbance of both body and space representation.

Child dyspraxia

Child dyspraxia displays a combination of body schema and space representation disorders, which is different from visual neglect. Dyspraxia is a non-lateral disturbance of skilled movements and space representation. Children with dyspraxia appear as awkward and clumsy; they have difficulty imitating other people's gestures, as well as naming or locating their own body parts (Lussier and Flessas, 2009); however, they also display enormous difficulties in copying geometrical shapes and orientating themselves on a map.

Apraxias

As opposed to dyspraxia, the term *apraxia* refers to acquired neurological disorders of skilled movements. Apraxias primarily affect the programming or organization of these movements and are not caused by sensorimotor or visual disorders. Apraxia may affect a variety of movements: symbolic gestures, routine movements involved in using the objects of everyday life, automatic movements (e.g., walking) or arbitrary gestures (e.g., during neurological examinations). As I have previously emphasised, any given gesture is always performed in a spatial context. Some particular forms of apraxia show the relationships between body schema and the management of space: some patients are able to use an everyday object but cannot 'mime' its use; in other words, they are unable to produce the same gesture when the task only consists of moving their hands in space (Buxbaum, Giovannetti and Libon, 2000).

Body schema disorders and psychopathology

In neuropsychological literature, body schema disorders are only considered to be cognitive disorders. However, some clinical data suggest that the psychological aspects of body schema disorders should not be ignored. Visual hemineglect is often associated with some kind of reticence, a lack of interest directed towards the left hemispace. This was noted by Bisiach (Bisiach and Luzzatti, 1978) in his princeps observation of a patient who was asked to imagine himself standing on the Piazza del Duomo in Milan and account for the surrounding monuments. The patient omitted several monuments on his left, but nevertheless did mention a number of them. Bisiach then noticed that the patient spoke vividly of the buildings located either in front of him or to his right, but seemed 'distracted' or even 'irritated' when asked to describe those he knew to be on his left. In addition, hemineglect is very often associated with characteristic types of subjective behaviour and discourse alterations, which have often been described in neurological literature.

Asomatognosia

Asomatognosia might be considered an extreme form of hemineglect, because asomatognosic patients ignore their left-hand side completely. They may even refuse to acknowledge the ownership of their paralysed hand, arm or leg when it is shown to them, instead telling the examiner: "It's a hand" or even "This is your hand". This disowning concerns upper limbs more often than lower limbs. The work of Hécaen and de Ajurriaguerra devoted to asomatognosia (1952) includes many similar examples.

Somatoparaphrenia

Asomatognosic patients may attribute the ownership of the paralysed hand to another person or even consider it as a separate human being (Gerstmann, 1942). The person in question can be a complete stranger ("they grafted another one onto me"), but most often it is someone close to the patient ("it is my husband's hand, he forgot it here when he left"). These disorders are not neutral from the subjective point of view. Some patients may give their hand a name or a nickname. Regardless of whether they personalise it, they can very often treat it with hate or scorn; hence the term "misoplegia" coined by Critchley (1962) to describe this behaviour. This spectacular form of somatoparaphrenia is rather rare, but minor manifestations are fairly common (for example, when an asomatognosic patient is shown his own hand by a neurologist and says "It is your hand"). Certain formulations uttered by patients regarding their paralysed hands should therefore not go unnoticed. For example, a patient may say: "I make sure not to look at it". When asked: "But why should you avoid looking at it?" the patient answers: "It gets on my nerves, I feel undermined by it, I always need somebody else because of that hand". In one study of patients' discourse, among the 70 patients interviewed during the first week after a CVA, 13 expressed some kind of personification of the hand (Morin, Timsit et al., 2003).

Anosognosia

Most patients with RBI and left-side hemineglect also suffer from left hemiplegia. Some of these seem unaware of their paralysis, even in cases of complete hemiplegia. This symptom was first described by Babinski (1914) and is mostly observed during the first days after a CVA. It sometimes results in the patient refusing emergency care (Katz and Segal, 2004). At a later stage of their illness, patients may try to minimise their motor deficiency; they may say: "all of that is sleeping" or "the arm is tired". Although they often verbally admit that they are paralysed, they seem unconcerned about this paralysis or its consequences. Not only do anosognosic patients ignore the therapists' efforts to make them conscious of their deficiencies, but they may also react in an overly sensitive manner, as if they felt persecuted by the rehabilitation team ("They say I am neglectful", "They want to treat me like a child").

The relationships between body schema disorders and subjectivity also manifest in children with dyspraxia and in adult psychotic patients.

Dyspraxia and personality disorders

Children with dyspraxia suffer from 'personality disorders'. This refers not only to the children's psychological reactions to their poor academic performance or their clumsiness (cf. Lussier and Flessas, 2009). According to Stambak, L'Hériteau, Auzias, Bergès and de Ajurriaguerra (1964), some dyspraxic children exhibit "pre-psychotic" symptoms; these are in fact precisely those with the most severe disturbances of body schema.

Schizophrenia and body schema disorders

Schizophrenic patients may also suffer from disorders of self-representation and sense of agency (Jeannerod, 2003; Jeannerod, 2009). Lallart, Lallart and Jouvent (2009) used virtual reality tasks to show that psychotic patients performed particularly poorly at tasks which disturbed the ordinary relationships between body and space, e.g., when the visual information from the right side and the left side of space were artificially reversed. In these experiments, the subjects stood in front of a screen where they could see their own image reversed, together with non-reversed images of moving targets. They were instructed to catch the targets, so that they had to use their right hand to catch targets in their left space and vice versa. Normal subjects find this task difficult, all the more so if the image of their trunk, i.e., their body axis, is masked. Unlike normal subjects, schizophrenic patients do not perform any better even when their trunk is visible. They also do not feel the virtual context as real, as 'present', the way normal subjects do. They seem to behave as if they were lacking some bodily cue that could connect the virtual situation or their sensations to their bodies. Some authors consider that for normal subjects, this bodily cue might be provided by the "efference copy" or corollary discharge (see Mathalon and Ford, 2008).

In summary, whichever body schema pathology we observe, in one way or another it is always related to a disturbance of the subjective body representation. In the following chapters, I will use the term *body image* to designate these subjective aspects of body representation.

References

Babinski, J. (1914). Contribution à l'étude des troubles mentaux dans l'hémiplégie organique cérébrale (anosognosie). *Revue Neurologique (Paris)*, *1*, 845–848.

Bartolomeo, P., D'Erme, P., Perri, R., Gainotti, G. (1998). Perception and action in hemispatial neglect. *Neuropsychologia*, *36*, 227–237.

Berthaud, G., Gibello, B. (1970). Schéma corporel et image du corps. *Perspectives psychiatriques*, *29*, 23–35.

Berti, A., Frassinetti, F., Umiltà, C. (1994). Nonconscious reading? Evidence from neglect dyslexia. *Cortex*, *30*, 181–197.

Bisiach, E., Luzzatti, C. (1978). Unilateral neglect and representational space. *Cortex*, *14*, 129–133.

Bisiach, E., Luzzatti, C., Perani, D. (1979). Unilateral neglect, representational schema and consciousness. *Brain*, *102*, 609–618.

Bonnier, P. (1902). Le sens des attitudes. *Nouvelle Iconographie de La Salpêtrière*, *15*, 146–183.

Botvinick, M., Cohen, J. (1998). Rubber hands "feel" touch that eyes see. *Nature, 391*, 756.

Buxbaum, L.J., Coslett, H.B. (2001). Specialised structural descriptions for human body parts: Evidence from autotopoagnosia. *Cognitive Neuropsychology, 18*, 298–306.

Buxbaum, L.J., Giovannetti, T., Libon, D. (2000). The role of the dynamic body schema in praxis: Evidence from primary progressive apraxia. *Brain and Cognition, 44*, 166–191.

Coslett, H.B. (1998). Evidence for a disturbance of the body schema in neglect. *Brain and Cognition, 37*, 527–544.

Critchley, M. (1962). Clinical investigation of disease of the parietal lobes of the brain. *Medical Clinics of North America, 46*, 837–857.

Decety, J., Sommerville, J. (2003). Shared representations between self and other: A social cognitive neuroscience view. *Trends in Cognitive Sciences, 7*, 527–533.

Dolto, F. (1984). *L'image inconsciente du corps.* Paris: Masson.

Dupré, E., Camus, P. (1907). Les cénestopathies. *L'Encéphale, 12*, 616–631.

Gallagher, S. (2006). *How the Body Shapes the Mind.* Oxford: Clarendon Press.

Gallagher, S., Butterworth, G.E., Lew, A., Cole, J. (1998). Hand-mouth coordination, congenital absence of limb, and evidence for innate body schemas. *Brain and Cognition, 38*, 53–65.

Gerstmann, J. (1942). Problems of imperception of disease and of impaired body territories with organic lesions. *Archives of Neurology and Psychiatry, 48*, 890–913.

Harris, D.B. (1963). *Children's Drawings as Measures of Intellectual Maturity.* New York: Harcourt, Brace and World.

Head, H., Holmes, G. (1911). Sensory disturbances from cerebral lesion. *Brain, 34*, 102–254.

Hécaen, H., de Ajurriaguerra, J. (1952). *Méconnaissances et hallucinations corporelles. Intégration et désintégration de la somatognosie.* Paris: Masson.

Holmes, N.P., Spence, C. (2007). Dissociation between body schema and body image with rubber hands. *Behavioral and Brain Sciences, 30*, 211–212.

Hübner, C.F. (1794). *Coenesthesis.* Halle, Dissertatio inauguralis medica quam preside JC Reil, pro gradu doctoris defendit.

Jeannerod, M. (2003). The mechanism of self recognition in humans. *Behavioural Brain Research, 142*, 1–15.

Jeannerod, M. (2009). The sense of agency and its disturbances in schizophrenia. *Experimental Brain Research, 192*, 527–532.

Katz, J.M., Segal, A.Z. (2004). Should thrombolysis be given to a stroke patient refusing therapy due to profound anosognosia? *Neurology, 63*, 2440.

Kerkhoff, G. (2001). Spatial hemineglect in humans. *Progress in Neurobiology, 63*, 1–27.

Lallart, E., Lallart, X., Jouvent, R. (2009). Agency, the sense of presence and schizophrenia. *Cyberpsychology, 12*, 139–145.

Lhermitte, J. (1998). *L'image de notre corps.* Paris: L'Harmattan. (Originally published 1939)

Lurçat, L. (1974). *L'enfant et l'espace. Le rôle du corps.* Paris: PUF.

Lurçat, L., Wallon, H. (1962). Espace postural et espace environnant (le schéma corporel). *Enfance, 15*, 1–33.

Lussier, F., Flessas, J. (2009). *Neuropsychologie de l'enfant. Troubles développementaux et de l'apprentissage.* Paris: Dunod.

Machover, K. (1953). *Personality Projection in the Drawing of the Human Figure: A Method of Personality Investigation.* Springfield: C.C. Thomas.

Mathalon, D.H., Ford, J.M. (2008). Corollary discharge dysfunction in schizophrenia: Evidence for an elemental deficit. *Clinical EEG and Neuroscience*, *39*, 82–86.

Merleau-Ponty, M. (2012). *Phenomenology of Perception*. London and New York: Routledge. (Originally published 1945).

Morin, C., Thibierge, S. (2006). Body image in neurology and psychoanalysis: History and new developments. *Journal of Mind and Behavior*, *27*, 301–318.

Morin, C., Timsit, S., Durand, E., Marchal, F., Manai, R., Perrigot, M., Pradat-Diehl, P., Rancurel, G. (2003). Discours sur la main, asomatognosie et héminégligence. *Annales de Réadaptation et de Médecine Physique*, *46*, 514.

Mukamel, R., Ekstrom, A.D., Kaplan, J., Iacoboni, M., Fried, I. (2010). Single-neuron responses in humans during execution and observation of actions. *Current Biology*, *20*, 750–756.

Nadel, J., Decety, J. (2002). *Imiter pour découvrir l'humain*. Paris: Presses Universitaires de France.

Paillard, J. (1999). Body schema and body image: A double dissociation in deafferented patients. In G.N. Gantchev, S. Morin, J. Massion (Eds.), *Motor Control Today and Tomorrow* (pp. 197–214). Sofia: Academic Publishing House.

Preston, S.D., de Waal, F.B.M. (2002). Empathy: Its ultimate and proximate bases. *Behavioral and Brain Sciences*, *25*, 1–72.

Rizzolatti, G., Folgassi, L., Gallese, V. (2006). Mirrors in the mind. *Scientific American*, *295*, 54–61.

Schiff, M. (1894). Cénésthésie. In *Recueil des mémoires physiologiques de M. Schiff, volume 1* (pp. 469–480). Lausanne: Benda.

Schilder, P. (1999). *The Image and Appearance of the Human Body: Studies in the Constructive Energies of the Psyche*. Oxon: Routledge. (Originally published 1935)

Scholl, K. (1926). Das raümliche Zusamenarbeiten von Auge und hand. *Deutsche Schrifte für Nervenheilkunde*, *92*, 280–303.

Séglas, J. (1895). Mélancolie sans délire. In *Leçons cliniques sur les maladies mentales et nerveuses* (pp. 282–295). Paris: Asselin et Houzeau.

Stambak, M., L'Hériteau, D., Auzias, M., Bergès, J., de Ajurriaguerra, J. (1964). Les dyspraxies chez l'enfant. *La psychiatrie de l'enfant*, *7*, 331–496.

Starobinski, J. (1977). Le concept de cénésthésie et les idées neuropsychologiques de Moritz Schiff. *Gesnerus*, *34*, 2–20.

Vallar, G. (2015). Spatial neglect. *Journal of Neurology, Neurosurgery and Psychiatry, 86*, e3. doi:10. 1136/jnnp-2015 311750.12. Retrieved on 28/2/2017 from http://jnnp.bmj.com/content/86/9/e3.4.

Zazzo, R. (1988). 1945: Découverte de l'imitation néonatale. *Psychologie Française*, *3*, 5–9.

Chapter 2

Body image

In the 1930s, once the notion of body schema had replaced that of cenesthesia, several disciplines – especially psychology of child development (Wallon, 1931), neurology (Lhermitte, 1939/1998) and psychoanalysis (Schilder, 1935/1999; Lacan, 2006a) – became interested in what might be called "body subjectivity".

Wallon: acquiring the notion of one's own body

In 1931, Wallon showed "how children develop the notion of their own body" (Wallon, 1931). According to him, children first treat their bodies as if they consisted of distinct parts, each having a life of its own: at 23 months, a child can therefore offer his toes a piece of cake. Between the ages of 6 months and 2 years, the child discovers his own mirror image. Unlike young chimpanzees, children remain interested in this image even after they have understood its fictitious nature. While looking at it, they make jubilant faces and gestures; they turn back towards the accompanying adult, whose image they also see in the mirror. Importantly, a child becomes interested in his body image at a time when his body schema has not yet been built, at a time when he does not yet have any spatial notions, such as for example the difference between right and left (Lurçat, 1979), and is unable to enumerate his body parts. Wallon (1931) considers this early recognition of body image as "the prelude to symbolic activity, through which the mind transmutes the sensory data in a universe".

Lhermitte: body image in neurology

In his 1939 work *L'image de notre corps* [The Image of Our Body], Jean Lhermitte (1939/1998) wrote: "At the threshold of our consciousness, each of us has an image, a three-dimensional schema of our body, which enables us to feel, perceive, and ultimately develop our actions towards ourselves and the world around us." Based on Wallon's work (1931), Lhermitte reminds us that our knowledge of the form of our body is acquired rather than innate. As a neurologist, he insists on this image being registered in the structures of the brain; most of his book is devoted to studying body image disorders caused by brain lesions, particularly right brain lesions. However, Lhermitte also writes (p. 144): "It would be useless to look inside the brain for some fixed and rigid apparatus that would uphold an image as variable, as charged with meaning and history, as our actual body image." What we should retain from this definition is that body image exists as a kind of form but that this form, which is "charged with meaning and history", cannot be reduced to either a postural model or a purely visual representation. In other words, representing one's body to oneself is not solely a cognitive performance. Under the term "total asomatognosia," Lhermitte reports observations carried out by Deny and Camus (1905) of what today we would consider psychiatric rather than neurological cases: Deny and Camus in fact describe psychotic depersonalisation or melancholic syndromes very similar to those observed by Séglas and his disciples, which the latter formerly attributed to disorders of cenesthesia (we see how difficult it was for a neurologist to think of the relationships between body representation and subjectivity). In the first chapter of his book, Jean Lhermitte devotes a whole passage to "the development of body image, as seen from the psychoanalytic point of view". He has in fact read Schilder (1935/1999) and has taken on the importance of the erogenous zones as the "framework for the development of the structure of our image". "It is easy to imagine," he concludes, "all the interest that Freud's disciples have been able to draw from these 'observations', which, although we cannot provide any assurances in this respect, we wanted the reader to be aware of." However, precisely what interest could be drawn from psychoanalytic observations was not so easy to imagine: for many years, psychoanalysts failed to come up with a coherent theory of body image.

Freud and narcissism

In his 1914 paper *On Narcissism*, Freud defined narcissism as the process in which the libido is directed towards, first, one's own body, and, second, towards the ego, thus establishing a relationship between the ego and the body: "Applying our distinction between sexual and ego instincts, we must recognise that self-esteem has a specially intimate dependence on narcissistic libido" (1914, p. 97). Freud notes that the development of narcissism dramatically changes the relationships between the human subject and his body: In the autoerotic phase of early childhood, every body part may be a source of enjoyment; after narcissism is established, only a number of specific areas remain erogenous, while the human subject also comes to love his body, and a 'unity' – the ego – appears. Freud considers the mechanism of this passage from enjoyment to loving one's own body a mystery: "We are bound to suppose that a unity comparable to the ego cannot exist in the individual from the start; the ego has to be developed. The auto-erotic instincts however are there from the very first, so there must be something added to autoerotism – a new psychical action – in order to bring about narcissism" (p. 77).

Schilder, Freud and the libidinal structure of body image

In 1935, Schilder (1935/1999), both a neurologist and a psychoanalyst, coined the term *body image* as distinct from the body schema. Schilder stressed that the nature of the body image was "optical" rather than simply postural and functioned as a reference for perceptual data. However, it was not reducible to the visual image we have of our body: "The image of the human body means the picture of our own body which we form in our mind, that is to say the way in which the body appears to ourselves" (Schilder, 1935/1999, p. 11) According to Schilder, the term *body image* "indicates that we are not dealing with a mere sensation or imagination. There is a self-appearance of the body. It indicates also that, although it has come through the senses, it is not a mere perception. There are mental pictures and representations involved in it, but it is not mere representation" (p. 11). Schilder divides his book into three parts: the physiological basis of body image, the libidinal structure of the body image and the sociology of the body image. In the chapters devoted to the physiological basis, he describes the illusions of the phantom limb, as well as the neurological disorders of body schema. Yet these chapters also contain descriptions of a variety of bodily sensations, specifically those arising from the body's orifices, which are not part of the body schema. Schilder systematically links these sensations to the satisfaction formerly derived by the infant from these parts of the body. He seems to find in these antecedents the origin of the erogenous nature of the body orifices; his analysis of the libidinal structure of body image refers to the libidinal investment of the orifices and skin, brought about by a variety of contacts, exchanges and irritations in the infant's life. Schilder thus presents himself as Freud's disciple, referring to the notion of erogenous zones – oral, anal and genital (Freud, 1905) – and reminding us that through physical disease, any part of the body can become libidinally charged. Although Schilder is familiar with the paper on narcissism and states that narcissistic libido is directed at the body image, he does not make the link with the question Freud asks in his paper, namely, what is the process that must occur in order to move from auto-erotism to narcissism? In the chapter on the physiological basis of body image, Schilder comments on a variety of organic alterations of body representation. He specifically wonders about the meaning of the mis-recognition of hemiplegia (anosognosia), a puzzling lack of awareness that is observed in some subjects who have suffered a sudden unilateral paralysis. Schilder considers both this type of anosognosia, which occurs after a right brain lesion, and the phantom limb illusion, as "psychogenic formations". These would be due to the psyche being unable to admit the sudden lack, as a kind of "localised organic repression". For Schilder, this type of organic repression and the neurotic repression proper are distinct processes, but they involve the same mechanism: "When I use the term 'organic repression', I wish to emphasise that we are concerned with a phenomenon that, on a structural level, repeats what is going on in other repressions in the so-called purely psychic level [. . .]" (p. 32). Such formulations resemble a *petitio prinicipii* rather than questioning the psychical symptoms caused by neurological lesions. On the one hand, saying that organic and neurotic repression both employ the same mechanism might imply that losing control over one's body or its representation is no different from losing any other libidinally invested object – which is far from self-evident. On the other hand, Schilder does not suggest any psychoanalytic understanding of anosognosia for hemiplegia. For example, when commenting on the relationship between left hemiplegia and anosognosia, he never refers to the point raised in 1919 by Ferenczi (1952), who emphasised the symbolic specificity of the left-hand side as the 'bad' side. Instead, Schilder proposes a half-psychological, half-physiological explanation: The fact that anosognosia concerns left hemiplegia much more often than right hemiplegia would be due to a lack of motor impulses towards the left side, a tendency related to the normal manual preference. It is also worth noting that although Freud came from a neurological background and was familiar with Schilder's work, he never showed any interest in the neurological pathologies of body image.

To sum up, throughout the 1930s, the process of investing the body libidinally largely remained an enigma, even to psychoanalysis. It only became possible to solve this mystery by considering the relationships between body image and the object. To Freud's question about the way in which human beings move from autoerotism to narcissism, Lacan's work gives the following answer: one, enjoying one's own body becomes limited to the areas involved in the link/separation with the Other,[1] i.e., the erogenous zones; two, the investment of other body parts is repressed in favour of the body image, which is erected and offered to the Other's gaze. The Other's intervention suggests that what is at stake is no longer just body representation: Lacan offers us a theory of identification rather than simply an understanding of body representation.

Lacan, the specular image and the object

In his 1936 paper (see Guillerault, 2003) entitled *The Mirror Stage as Formative of the I Function as Revealed in Psychoanalytic Experience*, Lacan (1966/2006a) showed how it is that the body image may become – to recall Lhermitte's expression – "charged with meaning". To do so, he starts from a rereading of Wallon's observations, which he understands in terms of the child moving from a fragmented body (real state) to identification with an image (imaginary state). This mirror stage or mirror phase is crucial in the process of the subject's identification, i.e., in the acquisition of what we call an identity: The subject identifies with an image (imaginary identification). According to Lacan (1966/2006a), identification consists of "the transformation that takes place in the subject when he assumes an image" (p. 76). Crucially, this image is the image of a totality: the whole body, standing upright and unified. In addition, the subject assumes this image for an Other: the adult towards whom the child turns and who designates and recognises this body as the body of a named child. Words, i.e., symbolic elements, are attached to the image. Lacan thus revises the Freudian terms of ideal-ego and ego-ideal (Freud, 1923), insofar as the former refers to the virtual form of body image (imaginary identification) and the latter to the symbolic traits representing the subject in the linguistic register (symbolic identification). This process makes the infant a human subject, who recognises his body as a whole, as similar in its form to the bodies of others; at the same time – insofar as he has been given a name – it becomes his own body, part of the family lineage and assigned to a gender. Lacan (2004/2014) called this complex structure the specular image (see also Thibierge, 2011; Thibierge and Morin, 2010). Specular image thus brings together three heterogeneous aspects that are intertwined, entangled together: the real body, its imaginary form, and its designation in the register of language (Lacan, 1966/2006a; Lacan, 2004/2014). Human beings normally remain unaware of this "knotting" and of the fact that they identify with an imaginary form. According to Lacan, the ego is thus basically characterised by what it fails to recognise; the petrifying and alienating effects of identifying with an image stem from this *méconnaissance*.[2] Insofar as the subject is unaware of the real and symbolic determinants of his desire, he tends to desire in rivalry with others and will resist any attempts at putting this image in question. In 1949, Lacan (1966/2006a, p. 79) writes about the mirror stage:

> This moment at which the mirror stage comes to an end and inaugurates, through identification with the image of one's semblable and the drama of primordial jealousy (so well brought about by the Charlotte Bühler's school in cases of transitivism in children), the dialectic that will henceforth link the *I* to elaborated social situations. It is this moment that decisively tips the whole of human knowledge [savoir] into being mediated by the other's desire, constitutes its objects in an abstract equivalence due to competition from other people, and turns the *I* into an apparatus to which every instinctual pressure constitutes a danger, even when it corresponds to a natural maturation process.

He returns to this double aspect of narcissistic *méconnaissance* – on the one hand, immobilising and deadly, on the other hand structuring (since it is part of the construction of the *I*) – again in his article on *Aggressiveness in Psychoanalysis* (2006c, pp. 92–93):

> But if the ego seems to be marked, right from the outset, by this aggressive relativity [. . .] how can we escape the conclusion that each great instinctual metamorphosis, punctuating the individual's life, throws its delimitation back into question, composed as it is of the conjunction of the subject's history with the unthinkable innateness of his desire?
>
> That is why man's ego is never reducible to his lived identity, except as a limit that even the greatest geniuses have never been able to approach; and why, in the depressive disruptions constituted by reversals experienced due to a sense of inferiority, the ego essentially engenders deadly negations that freeze it in its formalism. 'What happens to me has nothing to do with what I am. There is nothing about you that is worthwhile'.

Formulations such as "depressive disruptions constituted by reversals experienced due to a sense of inferiority" or "deadly negations that freeze the *I* in its formalism" seem particularly apt to describe the experience of our patients affected by the sequelae of a stroke.

It is also in terms of *méconnaissance* – of being unaware of the real body – that Lacan (1966/2006a, 1966/2006f) comments on neurological data. The fact that the child recognises the form of his own body very early on implies that at the time of the mirror stage, he in fact ignores his real neurological immaturity, especially in terms of motor skills. As an adult, not only is the subject unaware of the real organic functioning of his body, but he may also fail to take into account the accidental alterations of its form, as observed in the phantom limb phenomenon (see Ramachandran and Blakeslee, 1998).

However, the pre-eminence of imaginary identification also involves another form of misrecognition, namely of what the image owes – if only because it is recognised as a unity – to its symbolic determinants. That is the first important characteristic of the specular image. The other key characteristic is that the body image is libidinised: i.e., it is narcissistically invested. This means that, one, the subject is fascinated by the human form, and, two, that his body supposedly represents something for an other, and more fundamentally for the Other, i.e., that it is necessarily experienced – positively or negatively – as an object of desire (Lacan, 1966/2006b, 1966/2006e). This is what a body really represents and what is by definition irreducible to either a symbol or an image: what I represent for the Other and for his desire is precisely something I can neither control nor have a clear knowledge of. Solely this kind of intangible value can explain why a given body – sometimes one's own body – can have a particular attraction or appeal for a subject, when it could be considered as nothing but a variant of a standard form. And indeed, this form cannot be reduced to either a standard or an object 'simply' perceived because it also represents the Other's gaze, insofar as the subject questions his own ability to appeal to this gaze, to 'fit' the Other's demand or desire. This intangible x is what Lacan, following Freud (1905), names "the object" (Lacan, 2011, 1966/2006e); however, unlike Freud's understanding, Lacan's structural reading characterises the object in its relation to the erogenous zones. The erogenous zones are the areas of the body where the object loss manifests itself (Lacan, 1966/2006e): the mouth is where food and love are demanded from the Other, the eye and the ear receive the expressions of the Other's demand or desire through gaze or voice; the anus is the area to which the Other addresses his own demand. The object that suits this desire or demand can be represented in its four fundamental aspects: the breast, the faeces, the regard and the voice; however, it basically remains unattainable. This absence is designated by psychoanalysis as castration (Lacan, 1966/2006e). In addition, it is precisely insofar as it lacks this object that the body image can gain its consistency and that our own visible body or the bodies of others can arouse our desire. This lack, the precise coordinates of which normally remain hidden to us, has a kind of positive symbolic representation – the phallus, which must nevertheless be understood as a purely symbolic element, a signifier (Lacan, 1966/2006d). Any non-symbolic appearance of the lost object has disordering and upsetting effects; these range from Freud's sense of "the uncanny" (Freud, 1919) to depersonalization and include the many varieties of feelings of strangeness that have been described by classical psychiatry (see Thibierge, 2011). Hence it appears that the human subjectivity does not involve two components (the body and the psyche), but instead three levels or registers: (i) the object – the modalities of the subject's value and position in the eyes of the Other; (ii) the body image; and (iii) the *signifiers* representing the subject in the symbolic order.

This means that all our relationships to other people and the external world are structured by our singular ways of "lacking" the object and that this object has bodily antecedents: it has taken on its form in our bodily relationships (including the exchanges of gaze and voice) with the people we grew up with. Freud (1913) claimed that there was a link between the "anal character" and obsessional neurosis. Winnicott (1953) considered that the baby's comforter (the thumb or any soft toy, possession or vocalization) – an ersatz of the mother as an oral object – created an area where the future adult could begin to play and be creative. This building of a "space for lack" begins prior to the narcissistic identifications. Psychoanalysts who work with psychotic or autistic children have helped shed light on these "prehistoric", pre-narcissistic worlds. Their observations suggest that the way in which the baby's body is involved in subjective relationships goes far beyond autoerotic activities.

The body in clinical observations of infants and children

Since Winnicott (1953), the libidinal importance of the hand, fingers or thumb has been well known. Clinical observations by Françoise Dolto (1984) also show that the subjective body representation has little to do with body schema. For example, a little girl behaved as if she did not know how to use her hands or swallow; however, she accepted to take a piece of modelling clay in her hand and bring it to her mouth when Dolto told her: "You may take it with your mouth-hand."

Geneviève Haag (1985) has observed the use of hands in certain autistic children. Based on these observations, she claims that before the age of one, a baby may see its right side and hand connected to the mother and assimilate his left side and hand to some kind of self; the right hand may thus take care of the left one (see also Haag's work on "the Hands Theatre", 2002). As the body assumes an upright posture, this asymmetry may change, and the right side becomes invested with the phallic value. This clinical work shows us that some type of body representation – which is not limited to body orifices – is involved in a child's subjective construction from very early on, at a time when he is still neurologically immature and does not yet have any organised body schema.

Body image in psychosis

The presence of body image disorders in psychosis represents a point of agreement among the different traditions of psychiatrists and psycho-analysts involved in treating psychotic patients. For example, Priebe and Röhricht (2001), who work from a cognitivist perspective, have observed distortions in body representation in patients with chronic schizophrenia. They note that a "body-based psychotherapy" helps lessen the schizo-phrenic symptoms but has no impact on the body image disorders. This paradox is perhaps not so surprising, since the disturbances of self-representation in schizophrenia go far beyond simply a distortion of body representation. As the observations carried out by Gisela Pankow (1981) clearly show, what is lacking in psychosis are "the basic structures of the symbolic order which are central to language". The absence of these sym-bolic structures undermines the stability of body image.

Based on Cotard's syndrome, the work of Marcel Czermak (1986) offers an original reading of psychosis as both object and image pathol-ogy. Czermak speaks about the "passion of the object" (the etymologi-cal origin of passion is the French *pâtir*, "to suffer" or "be affected by"), suggesting that all humans suffer because of the object, in some way or the other. The Cotard delusion (Cotard, Camuset and Séglas, 1997) brings together a number of different symptoms: anxiety, ideas of being cursed or possessed, suicidal tendencies, self-mutilation, analgesia, ideas of having one's body destroyed, of having lost one's organs, body or soul, of being unable to die. Czermak reads these symptoms psychoanalytically; he emphasises the negation of the organs in the patients' discourse and the real dysfunction of the bodily orifices (mouth, eyes, anus) that they com-plain about. According to him, these complaints attest to a kind of fullness, a "lack of a lack" of the object, which disorganises the physiology of the body's orifices. In Cotard's syndrome, this too-present object is associated with the inconsistency of specular image. Cotard patients can describe their bodies as enormous or, on the contrary, as having shrunk to the size of a grain of sand. Such patients may thus be considered as "non-identified" ("The person of myself has no name," a patient answered when asked about her identity), deprived of the specular image ("I'm dispersed in space like things") and of an ordinary apprehension of the world ("The gaze is dead; I see colours and shapes, but it doesn't remind me of anything").

Thibierge (Thibierge and Morin, 2016) found the same association of a body image disorder and the intrusive presence of the object in Fregoli syndrome (Courbon and Fail, 1927). In this syndrome, the patient's body is invested and interfered with by a persecutory presence, which the patient discovers behind the figures and images of most of the people he or she meets. The patient designates this persecutor by a single name. In the princeps observation described by Courbon and Fail, the patient identified always the same persecutor (a famous actress) in the image of everybody she met. The actress was allegedly increasing her own beauty by using the patient's finger in masturbatory acts, i.e., by isolating a fragment of the patient body. In this process, the name, the object and the image appear separately. The Capgras syndrome – also called *illusion of the doubles* (Capgras and Reboul-Lachaux, 1923) – manifests another variation of this dissociation. In this delusion, the patients are convinced that their close relatives have been replaced by doubles or impostors. Capgras patients do not recognise the stability of the image of their loved ones and instead place importance on small details, which are supposed to make the *double* different from the person they used to know. The patient's own image is also destabilised. For example, when the patient described by Capgras (Capgras and Reboul-Lachaux, 1923) tried to list the specific traits that allowed people to recognise her, she gave a detailed description of her clothes, rather than her body or features. Her own name did not characterise her either, because she gave herself a whole range of family names. Today, Capgras and Fregoli delusions are classified under the category of the disorders of identification (misidentification syndromes). Originally, they were considered as 'false recognition' syndromes. Following Cutting (1991), Margariti and Kontaxakis (2006) note that all these syndromes in fact involve a difficulty in recognising *uniqueness*. Feinberg (2010) includes these syndromes among "the neurological perturbations of the self in which brain dysfunction creates a transformation of personal significance". According to these authors, Capgras and Fregoli syndromes, anosognosia and somatoparaphrenia are part of the same continuum (see also Dieguez, Staub and Bogousslavsky, 2007).

Identification, recognition, uniqueness, self – the variety of designations or theories show us clearly that these delusions pose a question to all the authors: what does being oneself consist of? What is involved in recognising other people as both similar to and different from us? Indeed,

I was standing, with that persisting romantic elation in me, as if I were a favoured fortunate person to whom everything was possible, I saw a stranger, a little, pitiable, hideous figure, and a face that became, as I stared at it, painful and blushing with shame. (p. 36)

Butler Hathaway's narrative wonderfully illustrates the fact that it is the gaze that is at stake, rather than visual perception or body representation. When speaking of her mirror image, the author does not describe its concrete characteristics at all. Instead she speaks of it as pitiful and ridiculous, as out of sync with the words she had previously used to think of herself ("healthy", "lucky"). When deciding to take a look at herself, the young woman is wondering about the image she offers to the Other's gaze ("I didn't want anyone, my mother least of all, to know"); she then cannot recognise her mirror reflection as the object of her mother's love. The Other's gaze is made out of words that had supported the narrator as a child during all those years she was confined to bed; moreover, though seemingly in conflict with her 'true' condition, they will continue to support her throughout her life as a woman. This example goes against the thesis developed by Goffman (1963), according to whom it is the norm admitted by a group that turns a handicap into a stigma. Instead, Butler Hathaway's account suggests that the defective body cannot be matched to an ideal of individual symbolic traits.

How to study body image using self-portraits

Drawing the human Figure has long been used as a method of exploring self-representation. While Goodenough and Harris (Harris, 1963) consider Human Figure Drawing as a test of the intellectual maturity of children, Karen Machover (1953) used such drawings as a projective personality test in children or adults who consulted her for psychological difficulties. Before asking the patients to draw themselves, Machover would first suggest that they draw 'a person', a man or a woman. Although asking somebody point blank to draw himself might seem somewhat abrupt (Bensalah, 1996), it is perfectly feasible to explicitly ask healthy, ill or disabled people to draw their self-portraits. Obviously this is made possible by the therapeutic context, which implies that the patient–therapist relationship is one of trust. At the same time, we also asked control subjects to draw themselves (Morin and Bensalah, 1998). These were approached, on one hand, in a geriatric outpatient clinic, where the patients were used to participating in various surveys dealing with ageing, and, on the other hand, in the rehabilitation department; in the latter case, inpatients' visitors and therapists were invited to participate as control subjects in a prospective study of stroke patients' conditions. We thus asked 98 normal subjects to 'make a drawing, a personal representation' of themselves. Asking somebody to draw himself – even just a human figure – necessarily mobilises the subject's questions regarding his body image and identifications. This was evidenced by the questions we received in return, and which we could hear as being addressed to the Other: "What do you want exactly? Is this a psychological test?" etc. The body that was then drawn on a sheet of paper manifested some of the traits of the specular image.

In general, the subjects did not try to represent their current physical appearance. In some cases, they drew a symmetrical, ideal-ego image: this was the case with a female medical student, who refused to use the pencil I offered to her and, using her own crayons, drew a portrait of a 'model child', an image that lacked nothing. Others drew their body wearing the insignia of their ego-ideal: an elderly man who never wore a hat nevertheless drew himself with – his father's – hat (Figure 2.1). The body they drew was sometimes 'transitively' shared with fellow creatures, as the one drawn by Mrs P, who was very surprised to see that she had drawn herself with only one breast (Figure 2.2); in fact, her best friend had just had a mastectomy. These individual observations confirm to us that the self-portrait can be a valuable tool for studying body image. However, an analysis of the whole series of self-portraits made by control subjects brings to light certain regularities or invariants; i.e., characteristics that are specific to normal self-portraits, which we are now going to discuss.

The normal self-portrait and its lacks

We find five main types of drawings (Figure 2.3): clothed figures, portraits made of stacked-on shapes, silhouettes, pictograms and naked portraits. When asked to show their right side on the drawing, the subjects ordinarily (9 out of 10 cases) point to the left side of the sheet, thus representing their bodies facing themselves. Most drawings (85 percent) give an impression of symmetry. Many are not only roughly symmetrical, but also

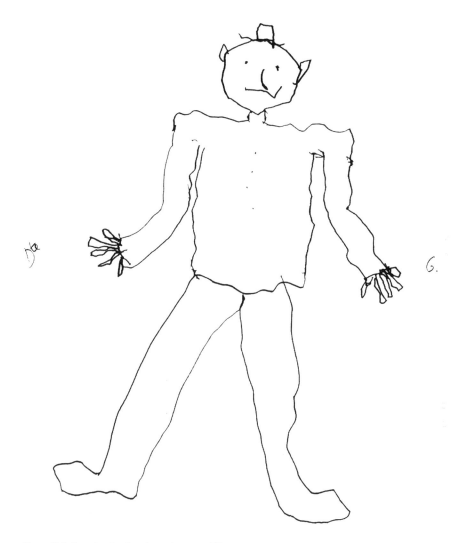

Figure 2.1 A retired school teacher, age 77
He has never worn a hat. His father, a village mayor, would never have gone out bare-headed. 'Dte' and 'G' were written by the patient to indicate the right [*droite*] and left [*gauche*] side of the figure.

complete (all body parts are visible in the position drawn); the figures are clothed, i.e., covered in narcissistic and socially sanctioned attributes. This confirms that in most cases, the response to the demand to draw one's own body is an imaginary representation.

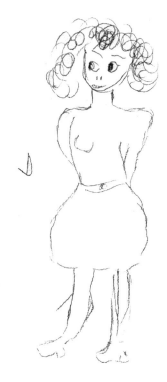

Figure 2.2 The wife of a hemiplegic patient, age 57
Afterwards, she realised that she had drawn herself with one breast only. She then told us she had recently visited a friend who had just had a mastectomy. The letter D [*droite*], written by the patient, indicates her right side on the drawing.

However, this ideal representation is neither without exceptions, nor without lacks. Firstly, facial features are not at all represented in six of the subjects (an observation that will be discussed when we come to Figure 2.6); secondly, the hands are drawn 'correctly' in only a few cases. It is rare (one out of eight portraits) for the hands to have all five fingers. Most often the hands are only sketched out (see for example Figure 2.3b, c, e, Figure 2.5a, Figure 2.6a, e, f); in one out of six portraits, both hands are completely missing (Figure 2.4). Likewise, even in 'complete' drawings, one or both hands may be missing or invisible, due to the position attributed to the portrait (Figure 2.5a and b). Although such representations seem realistic and natural, it seems important to us that as a result the

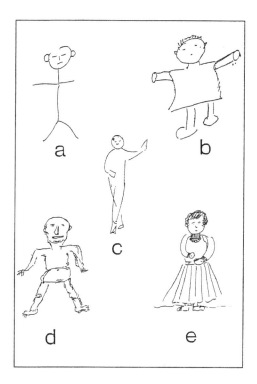

Figure 2.3 Typology of normal self-portraits
(a) Pictogram; (b) volumes; (c) silhouette; (d) a naked body; (e) a clothed figure

Source: Morin and Bensalah, The self-portrait in adulthood and aging, *International Journal of Aging and Human Development*, 1998, 46. Reprinted by permission of the journal and SAGE Publications, Ltd.

hands are hidden. The 'wrong' representation of fingers also contributes to making the drawing of hands problematic. Overall, the outcome is that the hands are drawn incorrectly (too many or too few fingers, one or both hands lacking) in 90% of normal subjects.

Karen Machover (1953) has previously observed the absence of hands in human Figure drawings by adults and children. While examining a total of 816 drawings made by students, Jones and Thomas (1964) also found that 16 percent of the subjects omitted one or both hands. These missing hands can be considered together with the comments made by the authors of the drawings: Whether they complain of their own clumsiness as illustrators or the difficulty of representing such an important organ as the

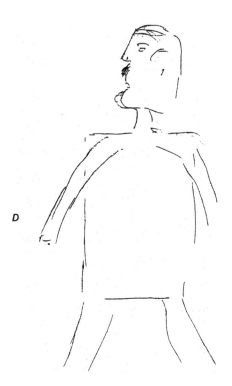

Figure 2.4 A self-portrait without hands by a retired school teacher, age 60
The letter D [*droite*] written by the patient indicates his right side.

Source: Morin and Bensalah, The self-portrait in adulthood and aging, *International Journal of Aging and Human Development*, 1998, 46.

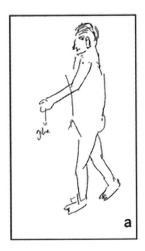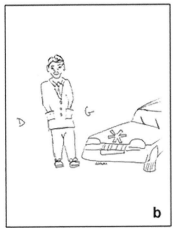

Figure 2.5 Self-portraits with one or two hands hidden
(a) A right-handed retired male engineer, age 75. Comments: "The right hand? It's disappeared, I can draw it"; (b) a male ambulance driver, age 36. Comments: "I have my hands in my pockets, because I'm not in my car." The letters 'D' and 'G' were written by the patient to indicate the right [*droite*] and left [*gauche*] side of the figure.

Source: Morin and Bensalah, The self-portrait in adulthood and aging, *International Journal of Aging and Human Development*, 1998, 46, as Figure 4, p. 56 and Figure 5, p. 57.

hand, these comments tend to suggest some kind of inadequacy vis-à-vis the required task.

> I didn't have a lot of time to draw and because I knew that I didn't know [how to do it] compared to my brother. . . . I also have a nephew who is a sculptor, he draws and he can draw characters just like that, something that I cannot do; I am really not very talented, I really have the least amount of talent in my family. [. . .] My father could also draw really well [. . .] well, these are people who after all know how to use a pencil; but my father didn't know how to draw faces [. . .] but my brother who's worked with stone also made faces, he would represent people. . . . My father didn't know how to do faces and neither do I.

In the drawing of the hand – or its absence – as well as in the comments that accompany it, we can therefore see a sign that each of us lacks something; in other words, a sign of castration. Likewise, here is the answer of a woman who was asked why she had left the hands, as she herself put it, "muddled":

> It's very difficult to draw hands. . . . In fact, in paintings I like precisely the hands and I think they are extremely difficult to draw. . . . As for me, I'm not doing anything, this is just doodling, these are not active hands, these are no hands at all, these are mittens, I mean, I think that drawing hands is just really difficult.

When people are asked to draw 'a hand', the result is quite different: 95% of the subjects draw a hand (the left hand in 75% of the drawings) with its five fingers. What we see here is a picture of the 'imaginary' hand (Freud, 1893), separated from the wrist by a straight line. In all cases, hands rarely leave the drawing subject indifferent. While drawing, many people say: "What am I going to do about my hands?" The comments suggest that there is indeed much interest in the hand. The patient above continues:

> I am very sensitive to hands [. . .] sometimes the hand is so elegant, it's superb . . . I don't like Léotard [the then–Cultural Minister] very much, but I think he has fantastic hands, the hands of an artist. I don't have beautiful hands. Recently I saw one of my nieces, who is quite

remarkable, I looked at her hands and thought: "What a pity! A woman of such calibre, it's not fair that she should have hands like that!"

The reader will notice the reference to sexual difference, a domain where there is always something 'not right': Léotard, whom the patient finds unpleasant, has beautiful hands, while she and her admired niece do not. In a similar vein (see previous citation), another woman emphasised how clumsy she felt compared with the skilful men in her family. These sexual connotations in comments suggest that the hand is one of the phallic signifiers.

We are indeed familiar with the hand's imaginary and symbolic "connections": the hand is an image of power, a symbol of the mastery exerted upon the world by mankind, as attested to by numerous expressions ('to have a situation in hand', 'to rule with a firm hand', 'to have the upper hand', 'to keep oneself well in hand', etc.). The hand is the insignia of power – for example, in the French kingdom the royal sceptre was called *la main de justice* [the hand of justice]. The power of the hand is also generative of life. The folklore around *mandrake*, the magical plant, illustrates the associations between the hand and the phallus (Leach and Fried, 1972, p. 477). From the Greek *mandragoras*, a mandrake is a root resembling in shape the human body; male and female mandrakes were supposed to be recognisable by their appearance. Mandrakes have long been thought to have powerful aphrodisiac and fertilising properties. While the English popular etymology combined man and drake, in French *mandragore* became *main de gloire* ('hand of glory'). In the popular tradition, the dressmaker's skilfulness in handling the needle was associated with sexual knowledge (Verdier, 1979). Yvonne Verdier reminds us that it is a prick on her finger that makes the sleeping beauty leave childhood and wait for her Prince Charming. The hand has thus the virtues of the phallus, which generates life. It also symbolises giving, exchange, alliance. In the expression 'to give one's hand', the hand is linked to the sexual difference in a symbolic register: in this case, it has to do with regulating the exchange of women (Levi-Strauss, 1949/2016), i.e., with the "circulation of the phallus" (Lacan, 1966/2006d). In addition, the hand is 'innervated' by all the words that refer to gestures, to the use of the hands both literally and figuratively: to handle, but also to hold, to take and their derivatives. As a metaphor, the picture of the arm appears in Egyptian hieroglyphs

(Champollion, 1836/2013), standing for the verbs such as to give, to drive, to have the upper hand, to calm, to separate, to reassure, and so on.

The signifier 'hand' is therefore part of the phallic series: the hand is celebrated as the glorious thing that, together with the erect posture, separates man from most other animals. However, the phallus also represents what half of mankind lacks, and is therefore also the symbol of lack (Lacan, 1966/2006d). Hence, the phallic signifier is the symbol of both power and lack. As seen previously in this chapter, the hand also has a previous history as a transitional object. As such, it has been lost as an object, and is marked by lack and desire. All these considerations suggest that in the process of drawing oneself, the hand signifies lack and castration (Morin, 1995).

The drawing subjects are much less reticent about representing facial features than hands. Although the eyes and the mouth are just as difficult to capture and draw as the hands, our subjects draw them without any hesitation. Some of them, regardless of their aptitude, readily talk about 'the gaze' or the 'little smile' they intend to show. However, the mouth and/ or the eyes are lacking in six of the drawings (Figure 2.6), whose authors are all over 65 years of age – the link between the advanced age and the drawing of a 'blank' face is statistically significant. Facial features do not seem to be missing from the drawings made by younger subjects (Jones and Thomas, 1964); this further suggests a relationship between older age and drawing a blank face. Five of these six subjects did not make any spontaneous reference to the absence of facial features.

This 'blank space' in their discourse contrasts with the vivid explanations related to the drawing of the hands. Only Mrs T (Figure 2.6d) explained why she had drawn a blank face, attached to a body wearing pretty clothes. She said that following the tragic death of her daughter, she had not been able to cry, or even to talk about her loss. Mrs T prefers to stay silent because "you are a prisoner of the words you have spoken aloud, while you are in control of what you leave unsaid". We could understand the blank face drawn by Mrs T as a neurotic symptom, a figurative translation of 'I have no eyes for crying; I suffer without being able to speak'. In elderly subjects, Clément et al. (1996) found a relationship between the absence of facial features from the image and depression. Mrs T's words might confirm such an interpretation. Given that these blank faces were drawn by six elderly subjects, five of whom were elderly

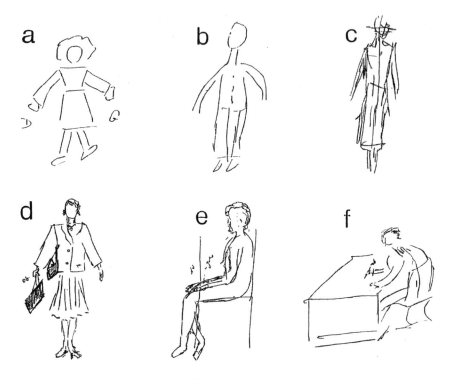

Figure 2.6 Self-portraits with a blank face
(a) A retired female real estate agent, age 78; (b) a retired woman lawyer, age 83; (c) a retired female decorator, age 84; (d) a retired female office manager, age 68; (e) a woman, age 72; (f) a retired male accountant, age 81.

Source: Morin and Bensalah, The self-portrait in adulthood and aging, *International Journal of Aging and Human Development*, 1998, 46, p. 58.

or very elderly women, we could also remember that according to Freud (1900), the eyes and the mouth may be displaced representations of the feminine sex. Finally, the non-representation of the eyes and the mouth – i.e., body orifices – might remind us of what Marcel Czermak (1986) calls, in his paper on the Cotard syndrome and its negation delusion (a negation of organs and body orifices), "the lack of lack of the object". Cotard-like syndromes are in fact commonly observed in elderly institutionalised patients (Ferrey, 1992), i.e., people who have lost the means of handling their world, of having meaningful exchanges with other people and who no longer occupy any imaginary or symbolic place in the society. Such patients (Ferrey, 1992) may claim that, contrary to medical results, their organs do not function properly. The declarations made by Mrs E (age 83) might be interpreted along these lines: Mrs E, who eventually drew herself as a kind of fashion figure, with no facial features (Figure 2.6c), had previously drawn a ball, explaining that she had "no shape anymore":

> My dear, you are asking me to do what? I would say [I am] like a ball, horrible now. . . . Before, I would have been a fairly normal girl, but now I have no shape anymore, it's quite another matter; I have no waist anymore . . . I prefer not to look at myself in the mirror. Now I am at an earthly level, inevitably because I exist, but I am preparing myself to be relieved of it and experience what will be outside my physical envelope. So I can't draw it for you, because I no longer have it.

The metaphoric value of the mouth and the hands

To summarise, far from showing us just an imaginary representation of the ego, the self-portrait can bring to light what Lacan calls the subject's lack-in-being [*manque à être*], under the guise of certain irregularities and deficiencies affecting the limbs and the facial features. These self-portraits thus show us, in very concrete terms, the metaphoric value of the different body parts, in particular the hands and the mouth. They confirm the lessons taught to us by the most trivial hysterical symptoms of everyday psychopathology, such as dysphagia (difficulty of swallowing) and paralysis. Just as common as these symptoms that "everybody can experience" (Israel, 2001), the mouth and the hands may be missing even from quite "normal" self-portraits.

Notes

1 Lacan distinguishes between two kinds of otherness: the other, that is, the fellow creature, whose form is fixed by identification to mirror image; and the Other, that is, the language determinations which constitute the subject, while being alien to him or her. Even before a person's birth, the Other in language registers the subject at a certain place and assigns symbolic marks to the subject. Being radically alien to the child (because of the incest prohibition), and the first to symbolically represent the child in her words and her relation to it, the mother is the first incarnation of the Other.

2 [Here and in the rest of this book, we leave the French *méconnaissance* in order to underline that it involves some kind of knowledge (*connaissance*) and is connected to the ego (*me* is a pronominal form of *moi*). Méconnaissance is "an imaginary misrecog-

nition of a symbolic knowledge (*savoir*) that the subject does possess somewhere"
(Evans, 1996, p. 109) – Translator's Note.]

References

Bensalah, A. (1996). Aimez-vous dessiner? *Cahiers de Linguistique Sociale, 28/29*, 283–289.

Butler Hathaway, K. (2001). *The Little Locksmith: A Memoir.* London: Aurum Press.

Capgras, J., Reboul-Lachaux, J. (1923). L'illusion des "sosies" dans un délire systématisé chronique. *Bulletin de la Société Clinique de Médecine Mentale, 11*, 6–16.

Champollion, J.F. (2013). *The Egyptian Grammar or the Principles of the Sacred Writing: The Foundation of Egyptology Translated for the First Time into English.* North Charleston: Create Space Independent Publishing Platform. (Originally published 1836)

Clément, J.P., Marchan, F., Boyon, D., Monti, P., Léger, J.M., Derouesné, C. (1996). Utilization of the Draw a Person Test in the elderly. *International Psychogeriatrics, 8*, 349–364.

Cotard, J., Camuset, M., Séglas, J. (1997). *Du délire des négations aux idées d'énormité.* Paris: L'Harmattan.

Courbon, P., Fail, G. (1927). Syndrome d'illusion de Fregoli et schizophrénie. *Bulletin de la Société Clinique de Médecine Mentale, 15*, 121–125.

Cutting, J. (1991). Delusional misidentification and the role of the right hemisphere in the appreciation of identity. *British Journal of Psychiatry, 159*, 70–75.

Czermak, M. (1986). Signification psychanalytique du syndrome de Cotard. In J. Clims (Ed.), *Passions de l'objet* (pp. 205–236). Paris: Editions de l'Association Freudienne.

Deny, G., Camus, P. (1905). Sur une forme d'hypochondrie aberrante due à la perte de la conscience du corps. *Revue Neurologique (Paris), 9*, 461–167.

Dieguez, S., Staub, F., Bogousslavsky, J. (2007). *Asomatognosia.* Retrieved on 11/3/2017 from www.researchgate.net/publication/281297088_Asomatognosia.

Dolto, F. (1984). *L'image inconsciente du corps.* Paris: Masson.

Evans, D. (1996). *An Introductory Dictionary of Lacanian Psychoanalysis.* London: Routledge.

Feinberg, T.E. (2010). Neuropathologies of the self: a general theory. *Neuropsychoanalysis, 12*, 133–158.

Ferenczi, S. (1952). An attempted explanation of some hysterical stigmata. In J. Rickman (Ed.), *Further Contributions to the Theory and Technique of Psychoanalysis* (pp. 110–117). New York: Basic Books Incorporated.

Ferrey, G. (1992). Le syndrome de Cotard et les négations fonctionnelles chez le sujet âgé. In *Délire des négations. Reprises 1992* (pp. 56–65). Saint Germain en Laye: éditions de l'AARPC.

Freud, S. (1893). Some points for a comparative study of organic and hysterical motor paralysis. *Standard Edition 1*, 157–174.

Freud, S. (1900). The interpretation of dreams. *Standard Edition, 6*, 339–626.

Freud, S. (1905). Three essays on the theory of sexuality. *Standard Edition, 7*, 123–124.

Freud, S. (1913). The disposition to obsessional neurosis. *Standard Edition, 12*, 313–326.

Freud, S. (1914). On narcissism: An introduction. *Standard Edition, 14*, 67–102.

Freud, S. (1919). The uncanny. *Standard edition, 17*, 219–256.

Freud, S. (1923). The ego and the id. *Standard edition*, *19*, 12–66.

Goffman, E. (1963). *Stigma: Notes on the Management of Spoiled Identity.* Englewood Cliffs: Prentice-Hall.

Guillerault, G. (2003). *Le miroir et la psyché. Dolto, Lacan et le stade du miroir.* Paris: Gallimard.

Haag, G. (1985). La mère et le bébé dans les deux moitiés du corps. *Neuropsychiatrie de l'enfance et de l'adolescence*, *33*, 107–114.

Haag, G. (2013). *Le théâtre des mains.* Paper presented at the 6th International Congress on Infant Observation following Esther Bick's method in Cracow, 2002. Retrieved on 2/02/2017 from www.genevievehaagpublications.fr/le-theatre-des-mains/.

Harris, D.B. (1963). *Children's Drawings as Measures of Intellectual Maturity.* New York: Harcourt, Brace and World.

Israel, L. (2001). *L'hystérique, le sexe et le médecin.* Paris: Masson.

Jones, L.W., Thomas, C.B. (1964). Studies on Figure drawings: Structural and graphic characteristics. *The Psychiatric Quarterly supplement*, *38*, 76–110.

Lacan, J. (2006a). The mirror stage as formative of the I function as revealed in psychanoanalytic experience. In *Ecrits* (pp. 75–81). New York: Norton. (Originally published 1966)

Lacan, J. (2006b). Remarks on Daniel Lagache's presentation: 'Psychoanalysis and personality structure'. In *Ecrits* (pp. 543–574). New York: Norton. (Originally published 1966)

Lacan, J. (2006c). Aggressiveness in psychoanalysis. In *Ecrits* (pp. 82–101). New York: Norton. (Originally published 1966)

Lacan, J. (2006d). The signification of the phallus. In *Ecrits* (pp. 575–584). New York: Norton. (Originally published 1966)

Lacan, J. (2006e). Subversion of the subject and the dialectic of desire in the Freudian unconscious. In *Ecrits* (pp. 793–702). New York: Norton. (Originally published 1966)

Lacan, J. (2006f). Presentation on psychic causality. In *Ecrits* (pp. 123–158). New York: Norton. (Originally published 1966)

Lacan, J. (2011). *The Seminar of Jacques Lacan: Book XIII: The Object of Psychoanalysis: 1965–1966.* Retrieved August 2017 from http://esource.dbs.ie/handle/10788/162.

Lacan, J. (2014). *Anxiety: The Seminar of Jacques Lacan. Book X.* Cambridge: Polity Press (Originally published 2004)

Leach, M., Fried, J. (1972). *Standard Dictionary of Folklore, Mythology and Legend.* New York: Funk & Wagnalls.

Levi-Strauss, C. (2016). *The Elementary Structures of Kinship.* Boston: Beacon Press. (Originally published 1949)

Lhermitte, J. (1998). *L'image de notre corps.* Paris: L'Harmattan. (Originally published 1939)

Lurçat, L. (1979). *L'enfant et l'espace. Le rôle du corps.* Paris: PUF.

Machover, K. (1953). *Personality Projection in the Drawing of the Human Figure: A Method of Personality Investigation.* Springfield: C.C. Thomas.

Margariti, M.M., Kontaxakis, V.P. (2006). Approaching delusional misidentification syndromes as a disorder of the sense of uniqueness. *Psychopathology*, *39*, 261–268.

Morin, C. (1995). La main en rééducation neurologique, réelle, symbolique, imaginaire? *Bulletin de l'Association Freudienne*, *62*, 15–19.

Morin, C., Bensalah, Y. (1998). Self-portrait in adulthood and aging. *International Journal of Human Aging and Development, 46*, 45–70.

Pankow, G. (1981). *L'être-là du schizophrène.* Paris: Aubier.

Priebe, S., Röhricht, F. (2001). Specific body image pathology in acute schizophrenia. *Psychiatry Research, 101*, 289–301.

Ramachandran, V.S., Blakeslee, S. (1998). *Phantoms in the Brain. Probing the Mysteries of the Human Mind.* New York: William Morrow.

Schilder, P. (1999). *The Image and Appearance of the Human Body: Studies in the Constructive Energies of the Psyche.* Oxon: Routledge. (Originally published 1935)

Thibierge, S. (2011). *Le nom, l'image, l'objet. Image du corps et reconnaissance.* Paris: Presses Universitaires de France.

Thibierge, S., Morin, C. (2010). The self and the subject: A psychoanalytical perspective. *Neuropsychoanalysis, 7*, 81–93.

Thibierge, S., Morin, C. (2016). Which identification is disturbed in misidentification syndromes? A structural analysis of Fregoli and Capgras syndromes. *Journal of Mind and Behavior, 37*, 1, 1–14.

Verdier, Y. (1979). *Façons de dire, façons de faire. La laveuse, la couturière, la cuisinière.* Paris: Gallimard.

Wallon, H. (1931). Comment se développe la notion du corps propre chez l'enfant. *Journal de Psychologie, 28*, 705–748.

Winnicott, D.W. (1953). Transitional objects and transitional phenomena; A study of the first not-me possession. *International Journal of Psychoanalysis, 34*, 89–97.

Chapter 3

The subjective effects of stroke

We might expect that stroke hemiplegia would raise the question of identity for the patient in ways that are similar to what Kathleen Butler Hathaway (2001) describes in the previously quoted passage. However, the brain origin of the hemiplegic disability necessarily renders the picture more complex. On the one hand, the generally accepted ideas regarding the psychic condition of stroke patients – i.e., their intellectual abilities have been weakened, they can behave childishly, etc. – may have stigmatising and deleterious effects. On the other hand, a stroke can cause highly specific psychic alterations, depending on the localisation of the vascular lesion.

Indeed, what we hear from patients in the rehabilitation unit is most often evidence of an ordinary narcissistic injury: most patients react to a stroke the way anyone struck by a sudden and disabling illness would. This will be discussed in further detail in Chapter 4. However, this is not true for all brain lesion localisations. Some may have specific cognitive and psychic effects, such as, for example, the right hemispheric lesions, which cause body schema disorders.[1] Such disorders specifically affect body image, hence affecting the individual's narcissism. This implies that after a stroke, we are likely to find two different subjective positions. In the absence of body schema disorders, patients react to the alteration of their ideal image caused by their stroke. These reactions do not appear intrinsically different from those of other patients responding to any other narcissistic injury. When the body schema is altered, body image can lose its coherence, and the person's narcissism – the love for one's own body – can lose its structuring function. These two kinds of discourse will be described in the following chapters.

Research methods

The patients' words reported in this book were gathered during clinical interviews. Most interviews were semi-directive. Some were audio recorded in full (with the patient's agreement), others were written down. When inviting the patients to speak with me, I introduced myself as a physician trying to understand what it was like to have a stroke from the patient's point of view. I also wrote down words I could hear directly from the patients during medical visits or consultations, or from the accounts related by their therapists during staff consultations. In all cases – whether these were unstructured or semi-structured interviews or simply everyday discussions – the patients spoke to people who were involved in their rehabilitation programme and keen on helping them. In semi-structured interviews, the following questions were systematically asked: Could you tell me what has happened to you? What is difficult for you now? What do you think of your paralysed limbs? How do you feel when you look at them or touch them, when you think of them? Have you ever had strange ideas about them (for example, that they might not belong to you)? Have you had any illusions of the paralysed limbs moving? Could you compare them to something or somebody? What do you imagine things will be like once you have left the hospital? How has your mood been? Have you had any dreams since your stroke? Do you think they have any relationship with the state of your health, your body or your hospital stay? During these interviews, the patient was invited to make a drawing 'that represented himself personally'.

Because people devoid of any brain lesions can also produce drawings with deficits, it would be difficult to formulate any a priori hypothesis about the links between, on the one hand, neurological symptoms or lesions and, on the other hand, the characteristics of self-portraits. This is why we used multivariate analysis, a descriptive statistical tool (Lebart, Morineau and Piron, 2000).[2] This kind of statistical analysis permits identification of differences and similarities among a set of objects, by analysing the variability rather than the frequency of a series of characteristics. We have thus examined a set of 308 self-portraits, among which 98 were drawn by control subjects, 75 by stroke patients with a left brain lesion, 86 by stroke patients with a right brain lesion, and 49 by patients devoid of any brain lesion but immobilised by a bone trauma or a spinal injury.

Each self-portrait was described in terms of the presence or absence of a series of traits: the hands and feet, the eyes, the mouth; the presence or absence of any accessories indicating age or disability (stick, wheelchair, arm brace, etc.); the presence or absence of clothes; the verticality and symmetry of the body axis; the positioning of the drawing on the sheet. As a first step, carrying out a Multiple Correspondence Analysis enabled us to determine the main discriminating variables, i.e., those whose presence or absence makes the portraits differ from each other the most. The second stage of the analysis, Hierarchical Classification, led us to split the portraits into distinct groups with shared discriminant characteristics. By examining these groups, we were eventually able to find out if the drawing subjects corresponding to a given group shared certain characteristics, such as brain lesion localisation, sensorimotor or cognitive deficiencies, age, sex, etc.

The specificity of brain lesions

This analysis led us to distinguish between three groups of self-portraits (Morin, Pradat-Diehl, Robain, Bensalah and Perrigot, 2003), which differ from each other in both their graphic features and in the share of normal subjects versus patients with right and left brain lesions among its members. The representation of hands (no hand, one or two hands represented), eyes and mouth (represented or not) proved crucial to differentiating the self-portraits from each other. Two groups exhibit characteristics that have already been observed in normal subjects (Morin and Bensalah, 1998). The most numerous group consists mainly of complete and realistic portraits in which both hands, the mouth and clothing are all represented. A second group has a high proportion of figures without hands and/or without a mouth. In both groups, the drawers are either normal subjects or patients devoid of body schema disorder, mainly patients with spinal injury or right hemiplegia and speech disorders. The third group contains 21 asymmetric self-portraits, which lack one hand or one foot and are inclined towards the right side of the sheet. Facial features and clothes are represented; in fact, many drawers insisted on drawing the clothes with meticulous detail. All drawers in this group have body schema disorders. Simply put, the self-portraits drawn by patients with body schema disorders are different from those drawn by patients without such disorders. The two following chapters are devoted, respectively, to the psychic effects of stroke in patients either devoid of body schema disorders (Chapter 4) or presenting such disorders (Chapter 5). In each chapter, the patients' self-portraits and speech are discussed.

A word of caution is necessary before the reader embarks on the following chapters, which present different, if not conflicting, clinical pictures, depending on the presence or absence of body schema disorders. They should be read as a didactic report on psychopathological research, the results of which cannot be directly applied to individual therapies. On the one hand, the fact that body image may lose its coherence in cases of body schema disorders does not imply that all body schema disorders inevitably result in such an alteration. On the other hand, the existence of two types of subjective positions in stroke patients must not lead us to dogmatically oppose two types of patients. In fact, a neurological body image disorder cannot erase the patient's psychic structure. The dialogue with each individual, whether or not he presents with body schema disorders, can only be fine-tuned based on what he or she says about himself and his or her body.

Notes

1 Body schema and body image disorders are of course not the only conditions to potentially alter the patient's discourse or behaviour after a stroke. In particular, the lesions or disconnections of the frontal lobe can also have behavioural effects, through various combinations of apathy and disinhibition.
2 The statistical software used was SPAD (Statistical Package for Augmented Designs, CISIA-Coheris, Suresnes, France). These tools are also included in commonly used statistical packages such as SAS and SPSS.

References

Butler Hathaway, K. (2001). *The Little Locksmith: A Memoir.* London: Aurum Press.
Lebart, L., Morineau, A., Piron, M. (2000). *Statistique Exploratoire Multidimensionnelle.* Paris: Dunod.
Morin, C., Bensalah, Y. (1998). Self-portrait in adulthood and aging. *International Journal of Human Aging and Development, 46,* 45–70.
Morin, C., Pradat-Diehl, P., Robain, G., Bensalah, Y., Perrigot, M. (2003). Stroke hemiplegia and specular image: Lessons from self-portraits. *International Journal of Human Aging and Development, 56,* 1–41.

Chapter 4

The psychological effects of stroke in patients without body schema disorders

Self-portraits[1]

As seen in Chapter 3, the self-portraits of the control group and the patients both with and without brain lesions can be divided into three groups. Two of these consist of drawings by patients without body schema disorders: the portraits in these two groups are vertical and symmetric. They differ from each other by the share of complete and realistic portraits including visible hands, clothes and facial features; this proportion is higher in the first of the two groups. In this group, half of the portraits have been drawn by normal (control) subjects, the other half by hemiplegic or paraplegic patients. This shows that the presence of brain damage does not necessarily prevent a patient from drawing himself just like anyone else would.

The second group of portraits mainly includes drawings with both hands, the mouth and/or clothes missing. These "poor" self-portraits, which may show a blank face and amputated hands (Figure 4.1) are drawn not only by patients with left hemiplegia, regardless of age, but also by patients without any brain damage (patients paralysed due to a spinal lesion or after having suffered a limb injury).

Two things should be underlined. One, these portraits do not reflect the actual asymmetry of the body alteration (whether the latter is due to a fractured limb or to hemiplegia). Two, the missing hands, mouth or eyes represent a striking alteration of the self-portrait, despite the fact that right hemiplegia, paraplegia or limb trauma are known to not affect body schema. However, we already know that the absence of these elements can be observed in normal individuals as well and is associated with ideas of insufficiency and incompleteness. It seems therefore logical to consider them as "symbolic and imaginary lesions", a way of representing

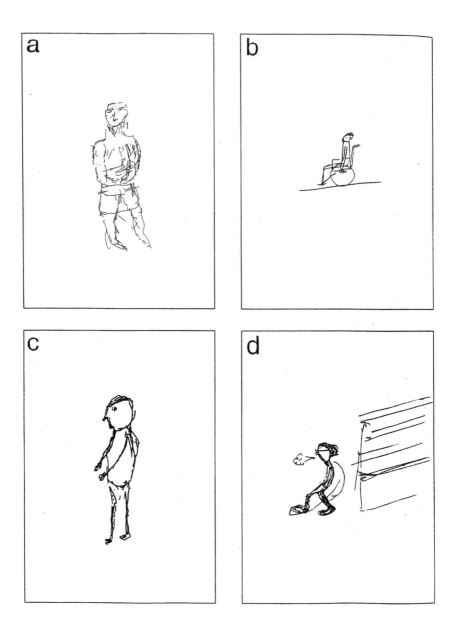

Figure 4.1 Self-portraits without a mouth (b, c) or without both hands and mouth (a, d), drawn by right-handed patients without body schema disorders

(a) A male physician, age 67, presenting with a right hemiplegia; (b) a male technician, age 42, presenting with a fracture of the pelvis; (c) a male surgeon age 69, presenting with paraplegia (spinal ischemia); (d) a male writer, age 40, presenting with traumatic paraplegia.

the individual's experience of helplessness and the damage caused to the ideal image by hemiplegia, as it would be caused by any sudden disability.

Missing hands

Stroke patients do not always comment on the absence of hands in their portraits. This silence is not easy to interpret, all the more so because many of these patients suffer from speech disorders. While such impairments do not necessarily prevent them from expressing their feelings or from understanding questions, they often impede complex or nuanced verbal expression. However, one patient made a surprising and clear statement (Morin, 1993). Mr A, a right handed patient age 74, had suffered a left-side pontine stroke and presented without any speech or cognition disorder.[2] His self-portrait (Figure 4.2a) shows him standing and unclothed. However, he does not seem naked, since neither his nipples nor navel is

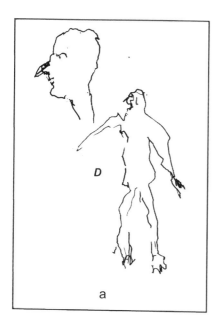 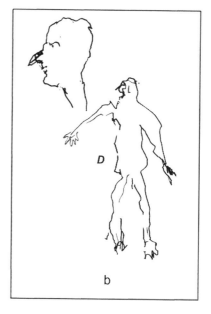

Figure 4.2 Mr A, age 73, right-handed, brain stem CVA, no cognitive disorders, no speech disorders
(a) The drawing of, first, the face and, second, the patient's whole body. The letter D written by the patient indicates his right side; (b) I myself added the right hand.
Source: Morin, Autoportraits de patients hémiplégiques, La psychanalyse de l'enfant, 1993, 14.

visible. The self-portrait is roughly symmetric, but the right hand is missing while the left hand is badly drawn. Only the nose is shown on the face. Mr A, a wealthy property owner, comments on the thinness of his arms in the picture: "I have nothing left. Before, I was plump and attractive." I then dare to draw what I think is missing from the picture, i.e., his right hand (Figure 4.2b). Mr A's reaction to my intervention is immediate and angry: in his wife's family he has once met, he tells me, a psychoanalyst, who produced unspeakable interpretations of children's drawings, a behaviour Mr A most strongly protests: "Me, I am all for decency. So I'd never have thought of speaking of anything sexual regarding what you have just drawn." However, there had been no mention of psychoanalysis during our conversation and I have not made any interpretations of Mr A's drawing. His reaction attests to the phallic value of the hand (in this case, the right hand), the command of which has been lost. Another clinical observation – this time of a female patient – runs along the same lines. Mrs D has been missing her appointments for the past two years. She has a very disabling hand paralysis and since her last appointment her motor skills have not improved. When she comes back, she does not ask to see her old physician, but then she spots him in the corridor and says: "If only I'd known that Dr X would be here today, I would have brought my eighteen-month-old daughter with me. He told me my hand was totally gone. I would have shown him! How do you make a child with a good-for-nothing hand?"

Lack of facial features

Likewise, patients rarely make comments about the fact of having omitted certain facial features; sometimes they make an unhappy grimace or a gesture. A paraplegic surgeon thinks that "what he's drawn looks like a bird's beak". He adds: "There's nothing human about it" (Figure 4.1c). The non-representation of the mouth could thus be interpreted as linked to the sudden and traumatising appearance of impairments and disabilities that isolate the patient from his social relationships, i.e., question his symbolic identity. This corresponds to the occurrence of similar behaviour in elderly patients, who can be confronted with the same questions, albeit in a more nuanced way.

Of course, the self-portrait is not the only way of accessing the questions of narcissism in stroke patients. Their reaction in front of mirrors, as well as what they say – and how they say it – when speaking of their situation, give us an insight into the image they have of themselves (Morin, Salazar-Orvig and Piera-Andres, 1993; Morin and Salazar-Orvig, 1996).

Mirrors and the gaze

There are many mirrors in a rehabilitation unit: from the reclining mirror above the wash basin in the bathroom to the full-length mirrors at the gym, including the mirrors in the elevators the patient is forced to use to move around the unit, either alone or accompanied, standing or sitting in a wheel-chair. Many patients avoid these mirrors; they do not adjust the bathroom mirror when having a wash and are reluctant to exercise in front of a mirror during the rehabilitation sessions. Mrs P says the following about them:

CM: And now, do you look at yourself in the mirror here?
Mrs P: Never. There is no mir . . . anyway, I'd have to get up, so, but in the room I can't.
CM: And when you have a wash, there is no mirror?
Mrs P: No – you do that . . . from . . . from memory.
CM: From memory! And would you like to see yourself in a mirror?
Mrs P: Oh well, I have seen myself. When I saw my face, I was not too pleased!
CM: When did you see yourself?
Mrs P: Oh well a few . . . a few weeks ago, I looked really unhealthy, I was all . . .

While Mrs P thinks she looks unhealthy, Mrs I finds her reflection "greyish"; most importantly, she does not recognise herself:

Mrs I: No use showing oneself to get . . . comments 'Ah she looks well, doesn't she?' and so on. Really! How well are you when you are in a hospital? They wouldn't keep you here if you were well. You see my point?
CM: So, you think you are not well?
Mrs I: Physically . . . um . . . but I don't look like the person I used to be. When I look at myself in the mirror, I don't recognise myself. Also because the mirror is slightly dark . . . slightly greyish . . . My reflection is greyish.

However, she finds it difficult to explain precisely in what way her image seems less familiar:

CM: What do you mean, you don't recognise yourself?

Mrs I: Oh yes, I've changed, I have my hair done any old way . . . um . . . well . . . so, that's not nice for a woman.

CM: Yes, yes, I understand.

Mrs I: That's all.

CM: Is it because your hair looks untidy that you don't recognise yourself?

Mrs I: Because of everything. My face, I lost a little weight . . . I am . . . you know how it changes a woman when she tidies herself up a bit.

As we see in the case of Mrs O, this uneasiness before the mirror may have to do with facial asymmetry, which patients never fail to mention:

> And . . . for many years, I had always been scared when I saw people in the metro, who had their face askew. [. . .] And when my husband came to see me at the hospital, he would bring me mirrors, he would bring me a mirror every day . . . so that I could see [. . .] and he told me: 'No, you've got nothing'. [. . .] When I'm asleep, I drool a little . . . things like that, but well, OK, my face isn't really deformed.

However, it is not only their reflection that patients "see" in the mirror. While a patient, Mr T is exercising in front of the mirror, and his physiotherapist asks him whether this kind of exercise is enjoyable or boring. Mr T answers that he quite likes it, because he thinks he looks "cute" in the mirror. However, a few days later, when I ask him if he likes working out in front of the mirror, he says that, in the mirror, he sees that "he is done for". What is at stake for him is indeed linked to the specular image, to identification and the narcissistic libido. It is the Other's gaze that questions the patient through the mirror reflection. In fact, as we have seen in the case of Mrs S ("no use showing oneself"), it is also the gaze of others that patients are afraid of. Mr D would like to look after his grandchildren, but only "if they don't see a grandfather who is completely un . . . senile". Rather than the gaze of others, we should therefore speak about the Other's gaze (see Chapter 2, note 2). Patients particularly dread being seen by those relatives they most value. Mr Y, who became paraplegic following a car accident, has been separated from his wife and children for many years. He now has no problem with them coming to visit him at the hospital, but he does his best to keep his girlfriend away ("Just think about it, a beautiful woman like her!").

Aggressiveness: the others' image

Some patients cast a jealous gaze at other people – caregivers or less disabled patients. Mrs A says to me: "Nothing would make me more mad – when I could not wal . . . put one foot in front of the other – than seeing people aged ninety-five or more walking ahead of me without any problem". Mr F, a hemiplegic patient, watches people pass him by and "rates them" in his mind. He explains:

> There is this blond woman there. When she's walking, it's wonderful, I'm in heaven, she holds her head high and her chest straight up. And then she is walking, she's clacking her heels and in my mind, I'm thinking that it's as if she's saying: "To hell with you! To hell with you!"

Self-image: seeing oneself "like that"

Questions regarding disability or paralysis often bring up representations in terms of image and gaze. For example, questions such as: "Did you know people who were paralysed?" and "Had you ever heard of such people?" often provoke answers with a shift in the expression: "I had seen some on TV or in the street", or "I'd never seen any". Before her stroke, Mrs I thought that being in a wheelchair was "the worst thing she could think of". She explains:

CM: So, before, you thought it was the worst thing you could think of?
Mrs S: Well, when I would see somebody in a wheelchair, to me they were finished, they were only half a human being. If the person doesn't have someone to assist them constantly, they are . . . really . . . I would say . . . really outside life, really outside, they can't do anything, [they] can't even go to the loo without having to tell someone.

But what is at stake is not only the patient's real gaze directed at non-paralysed others and his own mirror image, or the gaze his relatives directed at him. Let us listen to Mr E, a patient who found it difficult to see himself in the gymnasium mirror:

Mr E: Well, seeing oneself like that [. . .] at the beginning and, really it is true, there's no use beating around the bush: we are just wrecks, aren't we . . .

CM: Wrecks?

Mr E: Oh yes! All of a sudden – you are in good health, [. . .] you are normal, and then – snap! suddenly your life is . . . well . . . that's why . . . wrecks . . . you have a beautiful car on the road, and then, two hours later, it is being towed . . . they have to take it in a . . . Me, I say [we are] wrecks and I don't think I'm wrong. Perhaps it is a bit hard for some people, but me, I certainly am one.

Or Mr D, speaking of a friend who had a stroke: "It did not prevent him from living like that, dependent on someone [. . .] and I remembered it, when I saw myself like that . . ."

Being "like that", "in such a state", having "a disease like that" – these are all very common expressions among these patients. Using them avoids having to describe their problems. "As I've said, if I knew that I'd remain like that all my life, I would do anything to . . . leave" (Mr K). "I was like that and my wife had just had an operation" (Mr U). In a previous paper (Morin et al., 1993), we have shown that there is a significant correlation between these two discursive traits (referring to an imaginary gaze and designating one's illness as a condition "like that") and that they can be observed in all paralysed patients, whether they have suffered a brain or a spine injury. In other words, patients with a brain lesion are in the same boat as any victim of a serious and disabling accident. "Seeing oneself like that" might thus be considered as characteristic of the subjective reaction to disability.

Self-image and discourse: from I to one, the subject's subjects

The reader may have noticed that in the expression "seeing oneself like that", the grammatical subject is unspecified, even though the patient refers to the aspects of his illness that concern him most personally. This non-specification of the grammatical subject which designates the speaker reoccurs in many interviews. For example:

Mrs A: One becomes a bit like a child again.
Mr E: Well yes, you feel like a wet rag, don't you.
Mr Z: It was a disaster: feeling oneself stuck, paralysed, forced into a position of . . . dependency; suddenly feeling erased.

Mrs B (age 79, right hemiplegia due to a brain stem CVA) was the first to draw my attention to this way of handling the patient's "grammatical person". I invited her to speak with me by saying: "Well, I would like you to tell me a little bit about what this illness has been like for you." She answered:

> Well, it's unpleasant, of course, but one feels no pain, so I am always . . . I am particularly bothered because one is reliant on everyone, on all one's family . . . one has no independence or only very little and you always need somebody. So, I who always used to help others, seeing myself like that, it tires . . . it bothers me a lot. But after all, it shows one thing: all the love one is surrounded with. [. . .] I have many people around me and I hope that slowly . . . it will come back. It's hard because it hits you so suddenly . . . and without knowing why, see. [. . .] Anyway, one is . . . one thinks that one is nothing much [. . .] but what really bothers me is to be . . . a burden for everyone. I hope that soon I'll be able to at least walk. If one walks, one is saved, because, with the left hand, I can manage. [. . .] That's all I'm asking for. Because one can do nothing about it, one has to bear it . . . it's no use crying, moaning or anything . . . it does not get you anywhere.

When asked about that "one" she uses to speak of herself, Mrs B gives – as many patients do – a rational answer:

CM: At the beginning, you would often talk to me by saying "one does so or so", "one is": was this because . . . you wanted to give me information from a more general point of view?
Mrs B: Yes, me . . . I think that, what can you do, it's . . . the human being who is like that . . . it doesn't just happen to me . . . all

those who are like me, well, I think that perhaps they react as I do, or perhaps differently. Some people are . . . depressive. Me, I'm not depressive at all.

Implicitly, the position expressed by Mrs B ("it doesn't just happen to me") agrees with the position of linguistic studies looking at the use of non-specific grammatical subjects. These studies focus on situations in which the use of 'one' or 'you' includes the speaker in a group that, whether it is well defined or not, has at least potentially some kind of social reality (Viollet, 1988; Boutet, 1986). But this does not account for the way in which Mrs B shifts from the demand addressed to her (to speak about what her illness means to her personally) to an impersonal answer ("one is reliant . . . one feels no pain"). In fact, in all the interviews patients were questioned in a personal manner. Henceforth, they spoke about themselves personally, using impersonal means. This cannot but be related to how they see themselves.

However, when listening to patients, we cannot rely solely on our impressions. Before we try to characterise the relationship between image and discourse, we must describe, on the one hand, the precise way in which stroke patients handle the grammatical subjects when speaking about themselves. This is why I began to work with a linguist, Anne Salazar-Orvig, in order to carry out a systematic study of what linguists call *actantial schemas*. On the other hand, we also have to use a comparative method, in order to separate the traits characteristic of stroke patients (paralysed patients with a brain lesion) from those shared by all paralysed or immobilised patients. Therefore, we analysed the actantial structures (Morin and Salazar-Orvig, 1996) not only in the discourse of hemiplegic patients, but also in the discourse of patients hospitalised in the rehabilitation unit following a paraplegia (spinal lesion) or a serious bone trauma. This study allowed us to propose an interpretation of certain discursive behaviours in terms of a discordance between the patient's imaginary and symbolic identity.

Subjectivity and enunciation

From the linguistic point of view, the standpoint of the speaker does not manifest itself only through the descriptions, evaluations, or self-designations he may use, but also through the patterns that affect the ordering of his discourse or his coding strategies. Some of these patterns, not necessarily conscious,[3] concern the way in which the speaker uses and combines the different linguistic markers (mood, tense, personal pronouns). According to Benveniste (1974/2014), these 'shifters' (Jakobson, 1957/1990) are part of the formal apparatus of enunciation. This apparatus consists of 'empty forms' that become meaningful based on each concrete utterance. "When the individual appropriates it, language is turned into instances of discourse, characterised by this system of internal references of which I is the key, and defining the individual by the particular linguistic construction he makes use of when he announces himself as a speaker" (Benveniste, 1966/1971, p. 220). Benveniste thus considers the formal apparatus of enunciation as a manifestation of 'subjectivity in language'. Personal pronouns are among the 'Hobson's choices' in language, but they offer a range of units and effects of meaning which suggest different investments or semantic sets (Salazar-Orvig, 1999). In Indo-European languages, the first-person pronoun designates both the speaker and the person about whom something is being said. But other linguistic forms may occupy this place: when speaking of himself, the speaker can use *we, one, you*, or even make somebody else speak in his place. Using such forms has not the same value as using the first-person pronoun. However, the meaning of such an enunciation cannot be found in either the presence of such or such pronoun or in the frequency of their alternations.

From I to one, which verbs?

In order to understand the logic of why patients slide towards the grammatical markers other than the first-person pronoun, we were interested in the verbs that are combined with these shifters. In fact, patients used grammatical markers differently depending on whether they were speaking about their actions (action verbs possibly modified by auxiliary verbs – to succeed in, to try, to want, to be able to), their current state (verbs such as to be, to remain, to live, to become), the processes out of their control (to fall, to fall asleep, to suffer, to recover, passive verbs), or psychological or discursive processes (to feel, to have the impression of, to think, to see, to hear, to realise, to like, to loath, to dread, to hope, to tell, to speak, to explain, etc.). Even though we looked at other verbs as well (Morin and Salazar-Orvig, 1996), the three categories of (a) verbs of action,

(b) psychological verbs, and (c) verbs communicating a state – processes that are passively experienced or undergone rather than mastered – are mainly involved in speaking about the key consequences of an illness (limited or impeded action, dependency, suffering, being rendered passive) and the thoughts provoked by this situation. More than 75 percent of the verbs used by paralysed patients fall into one of these three categories.

Several grammatical subjects different from *I* may designate the speaker. Such subjects include the generic *you* ("Sometimes when you are sitting in your room, you think 'my God, there is so much work to do at home!'"), the collective *we* ("We have difficulty staying clean in bed"), unspecified subjects ("It's hard to bear"), as well as using second or third person in reported speech ("I said: 'Ah, you are like mummy!" or "In the Intensive Care Unit I heard: 'Look, her heels are black.'"[4]). Other markers should not be ignored, such as the use of the third person to designate characters similar to the patient – hospital roommates or acquaintances who have had a stroke. These characters permit the patients to also speak of themselves ("It's the same for everyone: falling . . . on the spot . . . and then that's it, there's nothing, no reaction, nothing . . . and all of them elderly people").

The results of our study, looking at the combination of the grammatical subjects – either "non-personal" subjects or I – with the three types of verbs mentioned above, may be summarised as follows (Figure 4.3): In patients who became hemiplegic after a cerebrovascular accident (CVA), the verbs designating a state (to be, to remain, to live, etc.) and those denoting processes passively experienced or undergone were combined with proportionally less I-subjects and more 'non-personal' subjects than in other patients. The way stroke patients handle grammatical subjects should not be ascribed to a cognitive disorder due to brain pathology: Combining the passive-suffering-experiencing verbs with unspecified subjects is very marked in patients with brain stem lesions, i.e., devoid of cognitive disorders (Morin and Salazar-Orvig, 1996). The opposite is true regarding psychological verbs and verbs of action. Patients with spinal lesions or bone traumas prefer to combine "non-personal" subjects with verbs of action.

Grammatical subjects and ego-images

Combining the clinical observations and the linguistic analysis of discourse leads us to conclude that what hemiplegic patients suffer from is

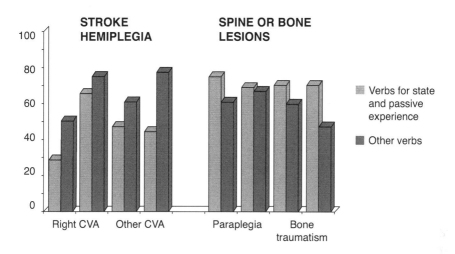

Figure 4.3 The actantial structures in the discourse of hemiplegic patients
The percentage of "I" grammatical subjects associated with (1) verbs designating a state (*to be, to remain, to live*, etc.) or a passive experience (grey bars) and (2) other verbs (black bars) in four patients who became hemiplegic after a CVA (bars on the left) and in four patients with spinal or traumatic bone lesions (bars on the right).

'seeing themselves like that', not being able to either name who or what they have become or recognise their image. In this context, to recognise can be also understood to assume that somebody is what he claims to be. We proposed to analyse these results based on the distinction between two identifications: the ideal-ego, an imaginary identification often supported by the body image, and the ego-ideal, through which the subject is recognised and recognises himself as bearing a given set of symbolic traits (Lacan, 2006a).

However, reading a linguistic analysis through a psychoanalytic lens means entering an area mined with confusions and "mistranslations". In fact, the words "enunciation" or "subjectivity" do not mean the same thing for both linguistics and psychoanalysis.[5] According to Benveniste, subjectivity is the position of a personal unity: "It is in the instance of discourse in which *I* designates the speaker that the speaker proclaims himself as the 'subject'" (Benveniste, 1966/1971, p. 226). "It is by identifying himself as a unique person pronouncing the *I* that each speaker sets himself up in turn as the 'subject'" (Benveniste, 1966/1971, p. 220). Lacan (1966/2006b) in turn argues that this subjectivity is a divided one and that, when listening to somebody speaking, a psychoanalyst must ask whether the speaker is uttering an enunciation (in which case the subject has no predetermined grammatical form or place) or identifying with his ego image. For example, among the sentences uttered by Mrs B (*I am particularly bothered – One is reliant upon everybody – That doesn't just happen to me – Some people are depressive – Me, I am not depressive at all*), we gave the greatest importance to the contrast between "I am particularly bothered" and "One is reliant upon everybody", two formulations which opened up the possibility of looking for regularities in the discourse of different patients, i.e., of statistical analysis. But, we could also consider the phrase "Me, I am not depressive at all" as a negation (Freud, 1925); in this case, the "subject of the enunciation" manifests herself in using the expression "not at all", which enables her to speak about depression without admitting to it.

We could assume that in the specific context of these interviews, in which a doctor-researcher offers patients the possibility of speaking about themselves and their illness, the resulting discourse comes from the ego. Because of the imaginary register it concerns, it is very likely to deal with the avatars of the person's narcissism. The alternation between two styles of 'self-designation' (I vs. unspecified subjects) calls to mind the two aspects of identification – imaginary identification (ideal-ego in Freudian terms) and symbolic identification (ego-ideal). This double position echoes the experience reported by Kathleen Butler Hathaway (2001), who used a hand mirror in order to be able to see her face when looking at her image. This kind of doubling seems to be condensed in one of the formulations quoted above: "I do not look like the person I used to be." We are therefore justified in making the link between the questions patients ask about their ego, their 'person', and what they have become, and the way they alternate between *I* and unspecified subjects when speaking about themselves. By using a linguistic form different from the first-person pronoun, the speaker tends to loosen the connection between his two positions – as the speaker and the person spoken about. This can be understood as questioning his ego consistency while simultaneously merging him with a group and thus blurring his singularity.[6] Displacing the stories or evaluations onto other characters further accentuates the distance between the speaker and the subject of the discourse. Lastly, we must remember – although from a strictly linguistic point of view, sex and grammatical gender are not the same thing – that in French, the non-specific pronoun *on* establishes a kind of neutral 'third person', which, being neither he nor she, would therefore be non-gendered. This could be seen as echoing the relative 'poverty' of many of the self-portraits, which are represented as unclothed, i.e., without sexual markers. The tendency of hemiplegic or paraplegic patients to use unspecified grammatical subjects when speaking of their illness can be linked to their pattern of designating their condition as being "like that" [*comme ça*]. Paraplegic patients, who preferentially combine action verbs with unspecified subjects might be particularly distressed by their inability to act, their motor deficiency, whereas stroke patients would question themselves about what they are, what they have become.

Narcissistic injury and recovery

This allows us to better understand the specificity of the subjective position of hemiplegic patients as opposed to paraplegics. The latter are 'persons with reduced mobility'. Although hemiplegic patients may be able to stand up and walk, they have suffered a brain lesion and are thus often considered as potentially senile; they have asymmetries, a 'crooked face' and often have lost use of one of their hands.[7] These characteristics – body asymmetry, loss of use of the hand – might constitute a stigma (i.e., a real mark suggesting a deviation from the symbolic order), which would make these patients consider themselves as intrinsically diminished individuals, rather than simply persons with motor deficiencies. Such a position nevertheless implies the continuity of the reference to a symbolic Other, as attested by the qualities of the dialogue with these patients. They are as if temporarily blocked, frozen in the mourning of their image, shattered by the changes affecting their bodies and functions. When asked about what they would like to do if they were able to walk, all patients therefore answer: "I would like to walk." A typical dream recurs in many hospitalised patients when they begin to recover: "I dreamt that I was walking." Sometimes 'walking' is part of a pleasant moment – for example, the patient is walking along the beach where he and his family used to spend their holidays. But very often the dream account is limited to the sole activity of walking. Indeed, such dreams generally occur when the patient is beginning to be able to walk on his own. We may wonder why patients dream of something that is already more or less happening in waking life – why should they have to dream about it? Yet we should remember that what the patient is recovering is the ability to move independently, rather than the ease and pleasure inherent to normal movement. Perhaps it is this loss that the patient feels when he becomes able to walk again. In addition, 'walking' might imply moving forward, with a well-functioning body (the French *marcher*, to walk, is often used in the sense of functioning or running smoothly). And in fact, these patients are still filled with a desire to move forward, to cope with their sequelae. It is worth noting that despite the various transferential relationships that connect them to their patients, this desire tends to remain hidden to the therapists.

For example, Mr X suffers from right-sided hemiparesis and sensory disorders following a left-sided stroke. An employee of an events management company, Mr X speaks about his profession using the expression *Je travaille dans l'événementiel*: due to the ambiguity of the French *événementiel*, the sentence can be understood either as "I am an events manager" or "My work has to do with day-to-day [i.e., inessential, banal] matters". Mr X says that his right hand is "a little child's hand". He is discharged from the hospital, having almost completely recovered. Then one day, he comes back to the unit, wearing a monk's habit. He has left *l'événementiel* (and now we understand that he used this word to indeed refer to factual concerns) to join a religious order, which requires its members to take a vow of poverty. Mr X used to be rather plump and found it hard to pass by a bakery without getting a croissant. His new life has freed him from these concerns, as he no longer has the money to satisfy his gluttony. This life change was directly caused by the stroke: according to Mr X, God has helped him to move forward into a new life, "like a little child". What may seem as a sudden crisis is perhaps related to the patient's long-term questions, which stem from him being an adopted child, with identity and filiation. About his life change, Mr X says: "On this path towards the Father, everything is joy and grace."

The paralysed body: absent from discourse, present as a transitional object

The discourse and self-portraits of the patients not suffering from a body schema disorder share a common trait – a silence regarding the paralysed body. When asked about the ways in which they can feel their paralysed side, almost all of these patients say that they notice the paralysis only when they try to perform a particular movement and fail. Although one of their hands is manifestly quite paralysed, hemiplegic patients will not mention it spontaneously unless it becomes a source of pain.[8] When asked explicitly ("What do you think about it? How do you perceive it?"), they describe it as a defective tool ("I can't do what I want with it", "When someone touches me, I can't feel anything"). For example, Mrs B shows me her hand and declares: "That does not move yet" [*Ca, ça remue pas encore*]. I inquire:

CM: What do you mean by "that"? You said: "That does not move yet".
Mrs B: How do you mean?
CM: You told me: "That does not move yet".
Mrs B: My hand, here.
CM: Your hand?
Mrs B: Well . . . It's completely dead. The hand, the wrist. Only the shoulder is working a little bit.
CM: Why do you say that your hand is dead?
Mrs B: Well, because . . . there is nothing . . . I don't . . . however hard I try to move it, it doesn't react.
CM: Yes . . . I can see that you are touching it a lot.
Mrs B: Well . . . Precisely, I try, because it tends to be . . . so I keep trying, I make it work [she laughs] as much as I can.

This dead, anonymous hand ('it') nevertheless manifests itself when Mrs B is speaking about her illness. In fact, as she is talking, the patient keeps vigorously rubbing her paralysed hand. When she is told: "You touch it a lot", she declares: "Yes, I play with it" (Morin et al., 1993). I have often observed this behaviour during the interviews with hemiplegic rehabilitation patients. Surprisingly, when I mentioned it during a staff meeting, it did not provoke any comments; Instead, the resounding silence was eventually brought to an end by the slightly meditative words of the head of the service: "Well, everybody tends to play with their hands, or produces some more or less automatic gestures when they are speaking". I was therefore forced to admit that these gestures, which are rarely mentioned in clinical literature (see, however, Weiskrantz and Zhang, 1987 and Van Stralen and van Zandvoort Dijkerman, 2011), were not recognised by the doctors. Could they be ignored or denied during medical examinations?

Or do they escape medical observation because they happen outside of examinations? Yet after our study was published, the clinical psychologist, the neuropsychologist and the speech therapists of the department told me that they had in fact often seen such gestures in patients. Like the latter, some of these clinicians considered them a way of forcing the hand to exercise, a practice that the patients thought did not receive enough attention during their physiotherapy sessions.[9]

In order to better understand the circumstances under which these gestures appear, we recorded different types of conversations with the same set of patients, i.e., in different transferential situations (Condat and Morin, 2000). During each dialogue, the types of gestures were noted down by a second examiner. As an illustration, let us listen to Mrs L, age 50, who presents with right hemiplegia due to brain haemorrhage (a complication of hypertension). She and her adult daughter are both unemployed and living in a squat. The first fragment was recorded a few days before Mrs L was discharged from the hospital, while she was questioned by the head of the department, Professor P, during one of his weekly rounds, which usually include several medical students. In the second conversation, Mrs L is talking with the Resident, who visits her daily. The third fragment is taken from an interview I offered to Mrs L, in order to talk about her situation.

Professor P's Rounds

Prof P: How are you doing?
Mrs L: Sometimes when I'm asleep in the morning I wake up and the back of my head always hurts.
Prof P: Has that been planned, that you would be going to a day hospital?
Mrs L: Yes, that's what they told me.
Prof P: It would seem?
Mrs L: Yes.
Prof P: Well, it's certain!
Mrs L: Oh really!
Prof P: For you it's always a "maybe"? Do you know what you're going to do there?
Mrs L: No, or . . . I mean, the same thing: physio [therapy], ergo [therapy] . . .[10]

Prof P: Everything went well during your weekends at home?
Mrs L: Yes, I mean, as usual. I was at home. Watching tapes. I should
            go out, but . . . I'm not very confident. I should try one day. I go
            out of the hospital . . . in the hospital.[11]
Prof P: You're going to get quite well?
Mrs L: Yes.[turning to a student] Did I answer well?

During this visit, Mrs L does not play with her hand at all. She is sitting
in her armchair, swinging her left leg (a small, rhythmical movement), and
she hangs her head down several times. She tries hard to 'answer well'.
The clinician's abrupt questions, which assess her current state and performance, turn the conversation into a dialogue aimed specifically at
establishing a decision, a prognosis, a *sentence* regarding Mrs L's future.

The Resident's Rounds

R: Have you been told to work on the right hand?
Mrs L: Yes. [Mrs L moves her right hand] Except for the difficult things,
            then I use my left hand.
R: Are you able to write with your right hand?
Mrs L: Yes [she mimics the gesture]
R: And with the left one?
Mrs L: Less so.

Mrs L mimics writing with her left hand, then she writes "I am healthy"
with her right hand.

Mrs L: I can't manage to do my hair properly. I usually brush my teeth
            with my left hand. And my head hurts.

Based on her complaint, the Resident then examines Mrs L.

R: Well, it's neuralgia. It's nothing serious.
Mrs L: I don't know. It's odd because it doesn't go away.
R: What doesn't go away?
Mrs L: This thing back here. I was at Claude Bernard [Hospital] for six
            months because I always had a headache. They found nothing.
            So . . . when do I go home?

This time it is Mrs L who is asking the questions ("When do I go home?") and declares, writing with her right hand, "I am healthy". But she eludes the main issue: to what extent is her disability compatible with her precarious lifestyle? She never asks questions about either her recovery or her future. Perhaps it is indeed the case, as we have seen in her conversation with the Professor, that her anxiety is expressed through her headaches – those headaches that will simply not go away.

Interview with Dr Morin

CM: Is there one side of the body that's bothering you?

Mrs L: No.

CM: I thought I had understood that in the beginning there was one side that was bothering you.

Mrs L: Yes, this one, a little [she points to the right side]. Things would not hold. It's difficult for me to wash my back, my head. In the beginning, I couldn't do anything because of the arm. It wouldn't hold. And the hand was like this [she squeezes her right hand]. Otherwise I don't have anything particular.

CM: Have you made any progress?

Mrs L: Perhaps with speaking. Now I can say words, before I couldn't at all. But I do feel something. At first I was wondering if I hadn't been paralysed, if I wasn't going to stay disabled. [Mrs L moves both her hands] The left one moves a bit more than the right one . . . [Mrs L silently squeezes her left hand with her right hand]

CM: And your mood?

Mrs L: My mood is fine. [Mrs L rubs her hands, moves them away from each other, intertwines her fingers] But it's not easy to have a neighbour like mine, who's crying all the time. I can't sleep at night. She snores, coughs . . . It's not clear how it happened. They've told me [it was] cardio-vascular. Maybe I was eating too much. An artery bursts, it seems. I wasn't stressed, but tired. Yes, tired all the time.

CM: You were tired because of your work?

Mrs L: I was unemployed. [Mrs L caresses her right hand with her left hand] Finding work – yes, that's difficult. I had a tension. That's true, that. They gave me half an aldactazine, but I guess it didn't work.

Mrs L touches her hand at the very moment when the discussion turns to her job, her main problem: "Yes, that's difficult". In other words, the patient is caressing her hand while talking about her most painful issue – a comforting gesture, which reminds us of Winnicott's (1953) transitional object.

To sum up, the patients who do not suffer from body schema disorders do not talk about the reality of their paralysed body very much, even though they may play with their paralysed hand. However, their words and self-portraits outline the non-gendered and impersonal form of a shaken and wavering ego.

Notes

1 The findings of this research have been previously published in Morin, Pradat-Diehl, Robain, Bensalah and Perrigot (2003).
2 Unlike hemispheric lesions, lesions in the posterior part of encephala (bulb, protuberance, cerebral peduncles and cerebellum) do not usually cause cognitive impairment.
3 The choice of personal pronouns [such as the alternation between *je* and *on* in French] is perhaps not always an unconscious operation, as illustrated by the following example. A patient relates his reaction immediately after breaking his knee: "So, the accident, well, it was not a disaster, in the sense that . . . when one was hit by the car . . . well it logically followed, it was not unexpected when one . . . um . . . I found myself on the ground, well the . . . what one immediately looked at was whether the toes could move, the ankle could move, then one noticed that it was at the knee that there was no movement anymore. Well, so one thought: 'it's here . . . there's some damage, and that's it', but it wasn't a panic, right . . . let's say that it was almost unavoidable, well, one thought: 'oh well, it's part of the job.'" The psychology student interviewing the patient then asks: "When you say 'one', who do you mean?" The patient answers: "One is me. Because – it's a thing I've often explained – because I had a father who always was very egocentric, we used to call him 'Mr I', so contrary to this I would say 'one' when speaking of myself.
4 [Meaning, she has got bed sores – Translator's Note]
5 To illustrate the difficulties of using the terms *subjectivity* and *enunciation* outside their linguistic or psychoanalytic context, we can look at the example of two contrasting fragments, one from the work of the writer Georges Perec, the other from a psychoanalytic article. In the first example, Perec (1990) is trying to convince his friends to become involved in the creation of a literary journal; as a former parachutist, he explains to them what it is like to jump from an aircraft. He says: "The fear was all the greater insofar as I knew what was going to follow [. . .] and as you move forward, you gradually lose your awareness of yourself [. . .] then, at a particular moment, one has doubts, there's nothing you can do about it, you ask yourself – well, it's not *you*, it's *I*. I have always asked myself why I jumped." The subject "Georges Perec" manifests himself not only in the movement from *you* (i.e., a member of a group of soldiers differentiated only by their rank in the file) to *I* ("I jumped"), from the present to the past tense, but also through the

reference to parachuting: When, as a little boy, his mother had to leave him to save his life, she gave him, together with his birth certificate, a comic book with the picture of a parachutist on the cover (Perec, 1993). The words of a psychotic subject, quoted by Marcel Czermak in *Passions de l'Objet* (2001), have a very different resonance. On the one hand, this paranoiac patient says to his son: "It is not because *one* has told you that you are Jewish that it is true"; on the other hand, in a letter concerning this same son, he writes: "*I* withdraw paternitie [*paternitée*] from him." In this text, the switching between *I* and *one* is not the evidence of a position of enunciation. Rather, Czermak shows that the subject confuses the real and symbolic registers, insofar he personally takes on something that depends on an external instance (paternity) and, at the same time, abdicates his place as a real father (*one* tells you). The extra *e* added to the French *paternité,* thus rendering fatherhood feminine, also shows the uncertainty of his subjective position.

6 In addition, in French the pronoun *on* etymologically derives from the word *homme* ['man'] (Bloch and Wartburg, 1994); we could therefore say that using *on* both blurs one's individuality and affirms inclusion in the community of mankind.

7 Fiszlewicz (1967) mentions the dread of asymmetry, which disrupts the "correct form" of the body image repeatedly: for example, a paraplegic patient states: "I couldn't have lived with an asymmetrical impairment."

8 Hemiplegic hand pain is often associated with shoulder and wrist pain, oedema and articular stiffness. Multiple factors may contribute to this complex neuro-rheumatologic disorder. Hemiplegic patients with sensory disorders may also suffer from neurological pain in their paralysed side, due to an imbalance in the central control of sensory perceptions. Such pain may be felt as chronic burning or crushing sensations. Patients can also sense brief painful flashes, like electric shocks.

9 The feeling that the hand is not being sufficiently retrained in fact corresponds to the usual lack of significant recovery, which means that therapists cannot suggest to hemiplegic patients any movements that would directly exercise their paralysed hand.

10 [*Ergothérapie* is the French expression for occupational therapy – Translator's Note.]

11 The patient makes a slip: Instead of saying that in the hospital she is quite capable of going out (for example, for a walk), she first says that she leaves the hospital: *Je sors de l'hopital*, and then corrects herself: *dans l'hopital.*

References

Benveniste, R. (1971). The nature of pronouns. In *Problems in General Linguistics* (pp. 217–222). Miami: University of Miami Press. (Originally published 1966)

Benveniste, R. (2014). The formal apparatus of enunciation. In J. Angermuller, D. Maingueneau, R. Wodak (Eds.), *The Discourse Studies Reader: Main Currents in Theory and Analysis* (pp. 100–140). Amsterdam: John Benjamins Publishing Company. (Originally published 1974)

Bloch, O., Wartburg von, W. (1994). *Dictionnaire étymologique de la langue française.* Paris: Presses universitaires de France.

Boutet, J. (1986). La référence à la personne en français parlé: le cas de "on". *Langage et société, 58,* 19–50.

Butler Hathaway, K. (2001). *The Little Locksmith: A Memoir.* London: Aurum Press.

Condat, A., Morin, C. (2000). Hémiplegie, papotage et tripotage. *Bulletin de l'Association Freudienne Internationale, 87*, 15–19.

Czermak, M. (2001). Identité . . . pas identité . . . supprimez-lui les excitants. De l'hypochondrie à la paranoïa, parenthèse et double boucle. In J. Clims (Ed.), *Passions de l'objet* (pp. 299–330). Paris: Editions de l'Association Freudienne.

Fiszlewicz, P. (1967). *Le handicapé moteur et la société*. Medical thesis. Paris: Faculté de médecine.

Freud, S. (1925). Negation. *Standard Edition, 19*, 235–239.

Jakobson, R. (1990). Shifters and verbal categories. In L.R. Waugh, M. Monville-Burston (Eds.), *On Language* (pp. 386–392). Cambridge, MA: Harvard University Press. (Originally published 1957)

Lacan, J. (2006a). Remarks on Daniel Lagache's presentation: 'Psychoanalysis and personality structure'. In *Ecrits* (pp. 543–574). New York: Norton. (Originally published 1966)

Lacan, J. (2006b). Subversion of the subject and the dialectic of desire in the Freudian unconscious. In *Ecrits* (pp. 793–702). New York: Norton. (Originally published 1966)

Morin, C. (1993). Autoportraits de patients hémiplégiques. *La psychanalyse de l'enfant, 14*, 140–147.

Morin, C., Pradat-Diehl, P., Robain, G., Bensalah, Y., Perrigot, M. (2003). Stroke hemiplegia and specular image: Lessons from self-portraits. *International Journal of Human Aging and Development, 56*, 1–41.

Morin, C., Salazar-Orvig, A. (1996). Paroles de patients hémiplégiques: discours et position subjective. *Sciences Sociales et Santé, 14*, 47–78.

Morin, C., Salazar-Orvig, A., Piera-Andres, J.B. (1993). L'hémiplégie après accident vasculaire: ce qu'en disent les patients en rééducation. *Annales de Réadaptation et de Médecine Physique, 36*, 3–17.

Perec, G. (1990). Le saut en parachute. In *Je suis né* (pp. 33–45). Paris: Seuil.

Perec, G. (1993). *W ou le souvenir d'enfance*. Paris: Gallimard.

Salazar-Orvig, A. (1999). *Les mouvements du discours*. Paris: L'Harmattan.

Van Stralen, H.E., van Zandvoort, M.J.E., Dijkerman, H.C. (2011). The role of self-touch in somatosensory and body representation disorders after stroke. *Philosophical Transactions of the Royal Society B, 366*, 3142–3152.

Viollet, C. (1988). Mais qui est "on" ? *Lynx, 18*, 67–75.

Weiskrantz, L., Zhang, D. (1987). Residual tactile sensitivity with self-directed stimulation in hemianaesthesia. *Journal of Neurology, Neurosurgery and Psychiatry, 50*, 632–334.

Winnicott, D. (1953). Transitional objects and transitional phenomena: The first not-me possession. *International Journal of Psychoanalysis, 34*, 89–97.

Chapter 5

The psychological effects of stroke in patients with body schema disorders

Patients with body schema disorders draw or talk about their paralysed body or hand in a highly specific manner.[1]

Self-portraits

As we have seen, the descriptive analysis of a set of both normal and recently disabled patients has helped us isolate a group of 21 drawings that greatly differ from the rest (Figure 5.1). These figures are asymmetrical, often leaning to the right, and they lack one hand and/or one foot. The facial features and clothes are shown; in fact, clothing can often be drawn with great meticulousness (Figure 5.1c). These characteristics contrast with those of the rest of the self-portraits, which always look symmetrical and vertical, even though certain body parts may be missing. The authors of these 21 self-portraits all suffer from disturbances of body schema and spatial representation. Hence we must take into account the problems that such patients may encounter while drawing. From the neurological point of view, asymmetries and deficiencies located on the left side of the page can be ascribed to left visuospatial hemineglect – indeed, hemineglect has been shown to manifest in different graphic activities. When drawing objects that come to their mind or copying pictures, patients with left-side neglect produce drawings with deficits on the left side (see Figure 1.2). However, the way our patients behave while drawing, as well as their comments and questions about their portraits, show that hemineglect is not the only issue at stake. For example, in 3 of the 21 patients, asymmetry and hemineglect were observed to diminish or actually vanish when the patient tried to draw

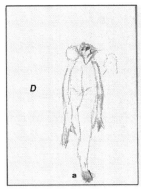
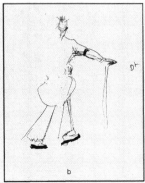
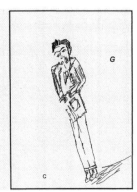

Figure 5.1 Self-portraits of right-handed patients with body schema disorders
(a) Mr J, age 50, graphic designer, left hemiplegia; (b) Mrs G, age 59, technician, left hemiplegia; (c) Mr B, age 69, engineer, left hemiplegia.
Mr J cannot yet stand up by himself; Mrs G has recently become able to walk by herself again; Mr B is still confined to his wheelchair six months after his CVA. The letters D, Dt and G have been drawn by the patients to indicate, respectively, their right and left side. Mrs G drew herself as seen from the back.

Source: Morin, Pradat-Diehl, Robain, Bensalah, Perrigot, Stroke hemiplegia and specular image: Lessons from self-portraits, *International Journal of Aging and Human Development*, 2003, 56, as Figure 6b, p. 23.

something that spontaneously came to his mind, i.e., something that interested him personally.

Mr S, age 45, a sales representative, has a Russian name which means "blind". Because of his anosognosia, Mr S does not believe his hemiplegia might prevent him from working the way he used to, often visiting up to 12 clients a day. His self-portrait is situated on the right side of the page; the Figure is missing its left arm and leg (Figure 5.2a). This is obviously due to left-side hemineglect. However, we should also notice that the missing arm and leg would not be located more to the left than the thigh and the shoulder, which are in fact shown in the drawing. In addition, when I point out that "Mr Blind" has drawn himself with only one eye, the patient adds another eye – a closed one! (Figure 5.2b). This closed eye can be interpreted in two different ways. We could consider it as a "slip of the pencil" (the equivalent of a parapraxis), suggesting that Mr S is trying to "close his eyes" when faced with the image of his paralysed body. This "left-side blindness" would therefore be a sign of the neurotic *méconnaissance* (see note 2, Chapter 2) of hemiplegia. But

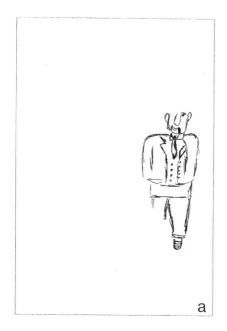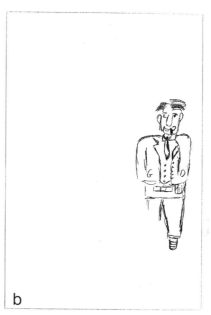

a | b

Figure 5.2 Self-portrait of a right-handed patient with body schema disorders, Mr S
(a) The first version; (b) drawing completed by the patient. The letters D and G were
written by the patient to indicate, respectively, the right and left side of the figure. This
allows us to see that the portrait is a mirror reflection of the patient.

Source: Morin, Pradat-Diehl, Robain, Bensalah, Perrigot, Stroke hemiplegia and specular image:
Lessons from self-portraits, *International Journal of Aging and Human Development*, 2006, 56.

we could also wonder whether the patient is not in fact drawing his own
name, which would attest to a confusion between the imaginary and
symbolic registers, in other words an unravelling of the components of
the specular image. This case is a good example of how difficult it is to
interpret psychic symptoms in patients with brain injuries: their symptoms do involve the patient's subjectivity, but they cannot be automatically interpreted in terms of the ordinary neurotic psychology.

Mr O, a right-handed writer age 58, suffers from left-side hemiplegia
following a CVA that occurred 3 months prior to the interview. His first
self-portrait (Figure 5.3a) is situated on the right side of the page, leaning to the left; it is missing the left-most side of the left arm and nearly
all of the left leg. Mr. O, who is a gifted pianist, then insists on drawing

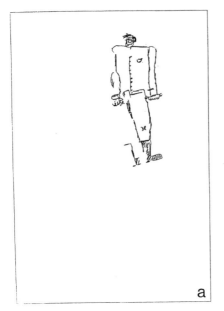
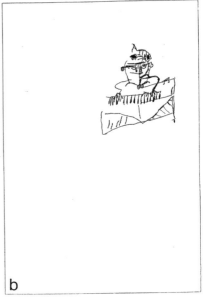

a   b

Figure 5.3 Self-portrait of a right-handed patient with body schema disorders, Mr O
(a) The first version. The letters DR written by the patient indicate his right side; (b) the
second version: Mr O playing the piano.

Source: Morin, Pradat-Diehl, Robain, Bensalah, Perrigot, Stroke hemiplegia and specular image:
Lessons from self-portraits, *International Journal of Aging and Human Development*, 2003, 56.
Reprinted by permission of the journal and SAGE Publications, Ltd.

another portrait, in which he is playing the piano. This second self-portrait
(Figure 5.3b) is less inclined and less asymmetrical: only the far-left edge
of the keyboard is missing, while both hands are visible and the asymmetry is mainly caused by the accentuation of the traits of the right half-face,
arm and hand.

Mr. G, 67, is a right-handed retired engineer and a keen amateur
painter, who suffered left hemiplegia five months prior to the examination, due to a haemorrhage on the left-side of the brain. His self-portrait
is disorganised (Figure 5.4a), since both arms are attached to the same
side of the body. However, Mr G then decides to draw a Figure he
would later like to paint (Figure 5.4b): a woman at the seaside, leaning
against a handrail. The figure's overall posture looks very much like

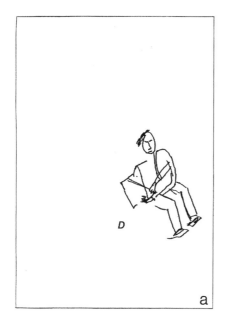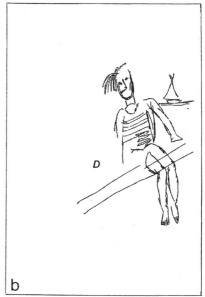

Figure 5.4 Self-portrait of a right-handed patient with body schema disorders, Mr G (a) A self-portrait; (b) a scene that Mr G would like to paint: a woman at the seaside. The letter D written by the patient indicates the right side of the Figure.

Source: Morin, Pradat-Diehl, Robain, Bensalah, Perrigot, Stroke hemiplegia and specular image: Lessons from self-portraits, *International Journal of Aging and Human Development*, 2003, 56.

the self-portrait, but the body representation is well structured. Mr G comments on his first drawing: "I don't know who that is, it's me. The important thing is the wheelchair, I spend three quarters of my time in it. [. . .] I have limbs, but I don't have a body that obeys me. I have an arm and a leg that I can't move – I can't mobilise them. But I see them as part of my body. But when I was in the neurology service, I had to think hard about how to connect my hand to my body. I said to myself: 'No, it's impossible. That hand is an extension of my body, it's just temporarily switched off.'" Mr G's body image is fragmented. His words (he has limbs but not a body) seem to describe the actual alteration of his body schema.

The unilateral deficits in these self-portraits are of course due to the disturbances in the patient's body schema and space representation. However, representing one's own body is not a neutral task and the different variations in the patients' discourse clearly show that the anomalies have a subjective meaning. This meaning is very different from that revealed by the portraits of patients who do not suffer from such disorders: the patients' decline and disability are represented; the alteration of body schema is made visible.

The patient's words

Patients with body schema disorders speak of themselves and their illness in much more pejorative terms than other patients with stroke hemiplegia. Patients with Right brain injury (RBI) often use expressions such as "a car wreck", "puppets on a string", "buffoons". They consider themselves not just "handicapped", "diminished" or "dependent", but also "childish", "fallen", "lame", "defaced", "half a man", "half-dead", "erased", "impotent", "out of order", "unable to express" [incapable de se manifester] or "unable to defend" themselves, "gaga" or "soft-headed" (Morin and Salazar-Orvig, 1996). Our 1996 study did not discuss the use of grammatical subjects in RBI patients. In clinical practice, it is not rare to hear patients, when asked about their current state, to answer using the formula *they say that*. . . . We could hear this as a form of anosognosia – as when a patient declares: "Everybody says that I have hemiplegia"; however, these patients can also say: "They say that I'm making progress", as if they were equally unable to take credit for their own recovery.

The paralysed body: present in discourse, subject to aggressive manipulations

The patients talk about their paralysed body in a very particular way. While most hemiplegic patients experience their paralysis only when they try to move, patients with body schema disorders can complain of a permanent heaviness or numbness of their left side (Critchley, 1953); they can comment on its swelling or colour. This form of attention to the paralysed hand, tinged with antipathy, might be a minor form of *somatoparaphrenia*, i.e., the personification of the paralysed hand as an external and hostile agent.

Patients with left-side hemiplegia play with their paralysed hand, but not at all in the same way as those with right-side hemiplegia (Condat and

Morin, 2000). During an interview, this is exemplified in the behaviour of Mrs C, a 52-year-old Spanish woman presenting with left-side hemiplegia and hemineglect:

CM: How are you?

Mrs C: Building puzzles makes my brain really tired. They make me do puzzles to see if my brain works as it should.

CM: Oh right, and so?

Mrs C: In my opinion, my brain is working well.

CM: And your mood?

Mrs C: I'm very tired – not sad, but tired [Mrs C plays with her paralysed hand, pinching and twisting it]. Of course, when I see that my limbs are working less well, I'm not so happy.

CM: Your limbs are working less well . . .

Mrs C stops playing with her hand.

Mrs C: My left leg hurts. But that is also because of the knee, because I've always had pain in my right knee. It's not just the paralysis. It's the arm that is the heaviest [Mrs C catches her hand again and twists it]. In the morning the hand is stiff, stiff, stiff. Once I get up, I try to make my leg walk a lot.

Mrs C stops playing with her hand.

CM: And your hand?

Mrs C: The day before yesterday I moved my fingers a bit, but not a lot. It's really stiff, really heavy. I have tons, tons of weight on my hand [Mrs C pinches her left hand again]. For me, the progress has been minimal. It's not like before. It's too soft, too heavy. Even at night it's sometimes too heavy. At night, I always put it on my stomach, like this, because otherwise it hurts too much. But even on my stomach it sometimes feels too heavy.

In this interview, Mrs C starts playing with her hand as soon as we begin talking about it, or when she tells me that she is not sad. As in the case of Mrs L, playing with the paralysed hand therefore occurs when the dialogue focuses on the lack or loss caused by the stroke. But unlike Mrs L, who gently caressed her hand, Mrs C's gestures are rather harsh and aggressive: She kneads the hand without any care. We should also note that she talks about the hand as of an anonymous, external and cumbersome object: "It's too heavy!" [*C'est trop lourd!*].[2]

Narcissism and body schema disorders

In other words, patients with marked body schema disorders cultivate a completely different relationship to their image than do other stroke patients. Despite their visible asymmetrical deficiency, the latter group maintains a stable, erected and symmetrical body image; they seem to undergo a classical mourning process in reaction to the loss they have suffered. They gradually abandon the neurotic *méconnaissance* which they have applied – together with everyone else – to their body and its alterations; step by step, they acknowledge the real loss. The question of the status of the paralysed hand remains suspended; it only becomes noticeable when the left hand begins to caress the right paralysed hand during a more upsetting part of the dialogue.

Contrary to these patients, patients with body schema disorders feel encumbered by the paralysed half of their body and, at the same time, experience their disability as a form of decline. Yet despite thus seemingly being in touch with the real gravity of their condition, they are at the same time anosognosic, i.e., unable to recognise the real consequences of their stroke. In addition, given both the aggressive gestures with which they manipulate their paralysed hand and the hostile tonality of somatoparaphrenia, it is difficult to speak about their narcissism – their self-love or the love they might devote to their body.

The somatoparaphrenia from which these right-hemisphere patients may suffer can help us understand the logic underneath the apparent strangeness of their discourse and behaviour. The relationship between RBI and the personification of the paralysed limb – which may also become inanimate, superfluous or cumbersome – is well established in clinical literature. However, the pathogenesis of these disorders seems to defy explanation. Some authors consider somatoparaphrenia to be a form of rationalisation (Halligan, Marshall and Wade, 1995), which would occur in reaction to the traumatising break-up of the body schema. Nevertheless, precisely because of the sense of oddity they induce, these productions seem quite contrary to what we would normally consider a rationalisation, and other authors have thus qualified them as "totally illogical" (Laplane, 1998). However, there are certain structures and themes that we repeatedly encounter in different patients; at the same time, there is an internal coherence underneath their apparent variety.

In the following chapters, this is illustrated by eight clinical vignettes, to which we then try to offer a psychoanalytic reading. In all these cases, the patients personified their hand to a greater or lesser degree. The four male patients talked about hemineglect in terms of body fragmentation or in terms of orality; the four female patients spoke about their paralysed hand as their daughter. These observations are then analysed in Chapter 6. Chapter 7 is devoted to a psychoanalytic reading of the right-hemisphere syndrome as a pathology of the relationship between the object and image, i.e., in terms of a pathology of specular image.

Notes

1 The findings of this research have been previously published in Morin, Pradat-Diehl, Robain, Bensalah and Perrigot (2003).
2 [The patient uses the pronoun "it" [ce] rather than the habitual "she", as the French feminine noun for hand, la main, would normally require – Translator's Note.]

References

Condat, A., Morin, C. (2000). Hémiplegie, papotage et tripotage. *Bulletin de l'Association Freudienne Internationale*, *87*, 15–19.

Critchley, M. (1953). *The Parietal Lobes*. London: Arnold.

Halligan, P.W., Marshall, J.C., Wade, D.T. (1995). Unilateral somatoparaphrenia after right hemispheric stroke: A case description. *Cortex*, *31*, 173–182.

Laplane, D. (1998). L'étrange en neurologie. *Etudes Psychothérapiques*, *17*, 23–32.

Morin, C., Pradat-Diehl, P., Robain, G., Bensalah, Y., Perrigot, M. (2003). Stroke hemiplegia and specular image: Lessons from self-portraits, *International Journal of Human Aging and Development*, *56*, 1–41.

Morin, C., Salazar-Orvig, A. (1996). Paroles de patients hémiplégiques: discours et position subjective. *Sciences Sociales et Santé*, *14*, 47–78.

Chapter 6

Case studies

Personification of the hand, broken up body, orality disorders, aggressiveness and transitivism

Hemineglect and the broken-up body[1]

I meet Mr E, a 69-year-old retired custodian, a few weeks after he suffered a right hemispheric CVA due to cardiac arrhythmia. His medical history includes lumbar and sciatic pain, which forced him to give up his previous job as a taxi driver. Mr E presents with left hemiplegia due to embolic ischemia, which struck him a month before our first interview. He also suffers from sensory disorders on the left side of his body and a severe left hemineglect in copying and cancellations tasks (see Figure 1.2). Mr E seems aware of his hemiplegia: he has been telling the occupational therapist that he could not do anything due to his left-side paralysis; he has explained to one of the externs that "it's all asleep" on his left side, so that he must use his right hand to move his left arm.

Conversation with Mr E

However, when I first suggest that he tell me what has happened to him, Mr E does not mention his hemiplegia at all. He immediately begins to talk; he keeps fidgeting in his wheelchair as I am pushing it towards the examination room. He talks about this wheelchair and about his pain, both of which remind him of his godfather: He would have never thought he would "end up like this", in other words, like his godfather, who "had both of his legs cut off and had pain in his toes". He describes his own pain (in shoulders and knees): "like ripping off the muscles, like peeling the bark of a tree". Since his godfather felt pain in the toes he didn't have, while Mr E feels pain in the joints he does have, Mr E wonders whether he should undergo an amputation. When he says this, he does not seem to be joking and appears quite unaware of the strangeness of his logic. I ask about the cause of his pain and he replies: "The attack split me in half. It starts from the head and then the pain spreads downwards, until it meets the chronic lumbar and sciatic pain and then blends in with them." Later conversations show that for Mr E, the back pain is a mark of his identification as a worn-out labourer. Crucially, Mr E does not spontaneously mention his hemiplegia; he only speaks about paralysis when he recounts the onset of his stroke: he fell off his chair and tried to crawl up. A neighbour said to him: "Don't try to move, your left side is paralysed," which he did not believe, until, he says, the emergency worker helped him up, making him realise that his left leg could no longer support his body.

How does Mr E feel about his left limbs? "They are heavy, they disturb me, they are dead weight." He feels his left hand 'flabby and sweaty,' 'sleepy'. He says: "I wish I could understand her; I have to bear her; she bothers me because she doesn't do anything." When asked if he has ever felt as if his hand did not belong to him, he answers: "Not really, but I wonder why she doesn't behave like the other one." He then speaks to his left hand: "Go and say good morning to your sister, take a walk together." He admits that since his stroke, he has often spoken to his hand in rather unkind words, as one would to a stubborn child ("Will you do something, you lazy-bones, you idle thing!"). When I ask about the future, Mr E says it is "a big question mark". He has heard about this type of illness before and knows that "it's tricky". Had he been younger, he adds, he would have been worried about being able to work again. He then chooses a more impersonal formulation: "There will be some improvement, one [on] has-seen worse!" When asked about his mood, he says: "I [Je] am in good spirits, I have no other major problems." He then explains that this is the way he has always dealt with his heart problems: "One [on] must have hope."

I ask about his dreams. Mr E speaks about dreams in which he "does a lot of things", such as "pulling on a rope, galloping". He used to have these dreams before his illness; they bring him back to his childhood in the mountains of Aubrac: He is running and jumping, he falls but does not hurt himself. These dream accounts could be understood as an example of what Freud (1925) designates as a negation, a denial of both the patient's prior sciatic pain (he falls without hurting himself) and his current hemiplegia (he gallops and pulls on a rope). In other words, Mr E knows – without knowing that he knows – that he is severely paralysed. Indeed, in their most optimistic form, his dreams represent a state that is now beyond his reach.

When asked if he has worries regarding his sex life, Mr E shakes his head: "It's as if all that has been erased from me."

Self-portraits

Mr E is asked to first make a drawing of himself, then to draw a human figure. Because of left hemineglect, in both drawings he uses only the right half of the page, regardless of its size: when presented with a double page, he only uses the right half; when given a single sheet, he only draws on the right side. He first decides to draw "his current situation" (Figure 6.1). In the picture, a head seen in profile, without any indication of the mouth, leans directly against the wheelchair; no other part of the body is shown. The whole Figure is falling towards the right. Behind the head, Mr E comments, "thoughts are evaporating." The hemineglect not only manifests in the placement of the drawing on the right side of the sheet, but it is also responsible for the missing spokes in the left wheel of the chair.

The patient is then asked to draw a picture of himself without taking account of his current situation. He uses the right sheet – the entire space of the page – to draw himself fishing in a stream (Figure 6.2). Again, the mouth is missing. The body is reduced to two vague strokes. The limbs are not shown at all. Stream fishing is seen as a specifically masculine activity, so that to identify it as a phallic symbol is not too risky an interpretation. More interestingly, there is a blank between the "body" of the fisherman and the fishing rod. This blank space could be related to Mr E's words: *it's as if all that has been erased from me.* The minimal character of the drawing clashes with Mr E's performance when I ask if there is anything missing from the picture, or whether he would like to add anything: in spite of his hemineglect, he then moves the pen towards the left edge of the right page and draws a very nice trout.[2] He also adds a "bird of prey" (more exactly, the right half of a bird of prey) seen in profile, oriented like the human figure.

This bird has no head and hence no beak, a parallel to the mouth absent from Mr E's portrait. Since both mouth and beak may be considered as sexual symbols (Freud, 1916), their absence, too, might be related to the "erasure" of sexual concerns voiced by the patient. The headless bird then

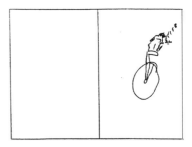

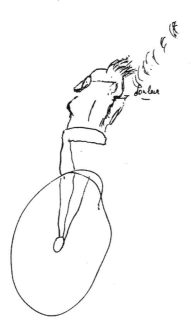

Figure 6.1 Self-portrait of a right-handed patient with body schema disorders, Mr E in his current situation. The patient wrote *douleur* (pain) just behind the head. The insert shows the position of the self-portrait on the double sheet presented to the patient.

Source: Morin, Thibierge, Perrigot, Right brain damage, body image and language: A psychoanalytical perspective, *Journal of Mind Behavior*, 2001, 22.

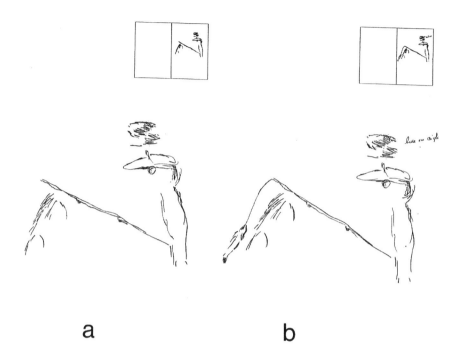

a   b

Figure 6.2 Self-portrait of a right-handed patient with body schema disorders, Mr E fishing:
(a) the first version; (b) drawing completed by the patient.
The insert shows the position of the self-portrait on the double sheet presented to the
patient.

Source: Morin, Thibierge, Perrigot, Right brain damage, body image and language: A psychoanalytical
perspective, *Journal of Mind and Behavior*, 2001, 22.

appears in subsequent self-portraits. For Mr E, it is associated with the
memory of damage caused by birds of prey on his parents' farm when he
was a child. These birds are known to attack suddenly, unexpectedly –
could this be related to the sudden onset of the stroke? In fact, according
to Mr E, the link between hemiplegia and birds of prey is in the claws – a
bird of prey has spurs [*ergots*] and claws [*serres*]. Mr E attends sessions
of *ergothérapie* (the French for "occupational therapy"), which in part
consists in using his hands in everyday activities – for example, to grip
[*serrer*] things. "I'm looking at a bird of prey flying above," he says, "it
has a prey in its claws, I don't know what it is holding, but never mind.
It's not *ergothérapie*, it's *ergot* [spurs]. Is it related," he wonders aloud,

"spurs [*ergots*] and *ergothérapie*?" Perhaps this also is a concern about the humanness of his paralysed hand (does he have fingers, claws or spurs)? Together with snakes, birds of prey are the patient's long-standing area of interest and he often talks about the excitement and fear they aroused in him as a child. Trying to destroy a nest of these birds, he once plunged his hand into a pile of dead snakes. Another time, he had to flee from an enormous grass snake.

Unlike my previous demand, Mr E finds my request to draw a random human Figure rather confusing. He prefers to draw Daladier (Figure 6.3),

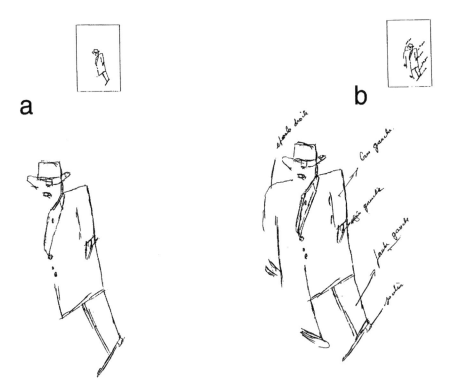

Figure 6.3 Mr E draws Daladier, the man who said "Peace is saved" while knowing there would be a war.
(a) The first version; (b) drawing completed by the patient. The left side is indicated by the patient. The insert shows the position of the self-portrait on the double sheet presented to the patient.

Source: Morin, Thibierge, Perrigot, Right brain damage, body image and language: A psychoanalytical perspective, *Journal of Mind and Behavior*, 2001, 22.

the French prime minister who signed the Munich Agreement and who declared, a year before the general mobilisation, to have "saved Peace". The mobilisation is among Mr E's most painful memories: he vividly remembers the young men with whom he was threshing wheat when the alarm rang. Many of them were later killed in the war. The left half of Daladier's portrait is missing. When I point out this absence to Mr E, he sketches out the missing limbs (Figure 6.3b), but does so without conviction and the result is still incomplete. In particular, he only draws the left shoulder and upper part of the arm, even though drawing the forearm and hand would not have required him to venture much farther to the left. Contrary to the first two drawings, here we have a structured body with a head, trunk and clothes, one hand in the pocket and one leg. The mouth is visible, but the eyes are hidden beneath a hat.

From the neurological point of view, Mr E should be considered to suffer from anosodiaphoria: his mood ("I am in good spirits") does not correspond to what he already knows about his illness (the future is a "big question mark" and had he been younger, he would have wondered about being able to work again). In this case, I would say that Mr E is not unaware of his hemiplegia, but the question of his paralysis never comes up spontaneously. Instead, his formulation ("The attack split me in half") indicates that his key problem is a disturbance of body image. When Mr E draws himself (as in the first two portraits), his body is either roughly sketched out or completely lost in the wheelchair, a symbol of decline. And, as we have seen, his body is also desexualised.

The disturbance of the specular image is localised; it does not affect the totality of the subject's psychic world. While his body is no longer invested with libido, other objects (trout fishing, nature) continue to arouse his interest and inspire his dreams and drawings. This corresponds to our experience of the discourse commonly maintained by patients with a right-side brain injury, who often describe their lost pleasures in highly vivid terms. Yet these pleasures seem to belong to another world, to which the patients expect to return by some sort of "trigger" [déclic] – a term used by a number of patients. Here, in the portrait of Mr E fishing, the rod is indeed "somewhere else" and a blank space separates it from the disabled body. Mr E hopes that "it will unjam", so that he may go fishing in the stream again. This expectation of some triggering mechanism, of "unjamming", cannot but remind us of its reversal: the break in the continuity introduced by specular identification. In retrospect, this break can actually feel as if moving from one world to another. In this sense, Mr E seems to have some insight into his condition.

As for the image of a body "split in half", it is attributed to another person, Daladier (Figure 6.3), who is supposed to have deliberately hidden the truth. These two aspects of the self-portrait (broken body, half-ignored body) are characteristic of the discourse of RBI patients, who can speak about their bodies with gloomy derision (Mr E later comments on another self-portrait by saying that he is "coming apart",[3] that he has not drawn himself but "a monkey or a hedgehog"), while apparently unaware of their real deficiencies. Mr E thus oscillates between two attitudes towards his specular image: As a whole body, he is "coming apart" and barely human (he looks like an animal); as a hemiplegic, he is split in half.

We note that the patient attributes the representation of this splitting to a character who is a *liar* – a choice that seems to indicate a kind of "active ignorance" of the left limbs. In the drawing of Daladier, the omission of the left half of the body, which is only reluctantly sketched out, raises questions about the kind of psychic mechanism at play. The highly revealing expression – "the attack that split me in half" – shows that there is no lack of knowledge (i.e., neither unawareness nor *méconnaissance*). On the other hand, the phenomena presented here, in particular the dreams in which he is catching hares or pulling on a rope, could result from repression. This repression is organised in a system which is specific to Mr E. Mr E does not simply assign to the Other what would be absolute knowledge; instead, he attributes to the Other the intention of hiding the truth. Just think of the hidden eyes in Daladier's portrait – the portrait of a man who, according to Mr E, wanted to conceal or ignore the truth. We must then ask: *What* is repressed? Mr E's attitude toward his paralysed hand can put us on the right track. Mr E speaks to his hand and reprimands it. He explains to me that when he experienced "the shock of having half of one's body not respond anymore", he thought of controlling his hand by addressing it the way his physiotherapist spoke to him during the physiotherapy sessions. "Of course it was stupid," he says, "my hand has no brain; there is only one brain." But he nevertheless continues in the same vein: "Now I don't speak to my hand as much, I wait for her to come to me." In any case, his way of talking to the hand is indeed not particularly therapeutic; it resembles the way one would speak to a difficult child. But when he is scolding his hand, the patient does not question his behaviour; he seems to be living in a fragmented body, a body consisting of pieces that can have an autonomous and even "personal" life. His hand is alien to him and its childish and undisciplined behaviour cannot but evoke the resurgence of a primordial link with the Other. Moreover, there is a slight feeling of disgust (the hand is "warm" and "sweaty"). Its personification is also apparent when Mr E explains that an arm-rest has been designed for his paralysed arm and he is constantly worried that his hand is not quite comfortable in it: "I'm always afraid that my fingers could be decapitated." In other words, the paralysed hand is no longer part of the body image.

This coexists with several symptoms in the oral realm. When I ask why the mouth is missing from his drawings, Mr E complains that he cannot taste food in a normal way. (His later comments reveal that this is hardly just a matter of physiology: A year and a half later, when he has returned home and says he can enjoy food again, he explains that hospital food was far from tasteless, but the meals were seasoned with "oriental spices"). Like many right-hemisphere patients, Mr E has lost the normal speech prosody (Joanette, Goulet and Hannequin, 1990.) The structure of his speech has changed: The normal pauses between sentences are lacking and the rhythm remains the same regardless of what he is saying. It is important to grasp the subjective coherence of these different facts – one way or another, they all concern the oral drive. The patient's symptomatology can then be read as an association of a disturbance of body image, the appearance of the object and a disturbance of the oral drive. This association shares a common structure with psychosis as it is typified by Cotard's syndrome (Czermak, 1986).[4]

To sum up, the patient's manner of speaking of his illness attests to a splitting of his specular image into, on the one hand, his 'half-injured image' and, on the other hand, his paralysed half-body, in particular his left hand, which appears as either a real object (Mr E finds it is "sweaty" or "warm") or an external character (it is "sleepy"). The association between disorders of orality and the fragmentation of body image is also crucial. The repression of the unmasked bodily antecedents of the object is at stake when Mr E draws Daladier (or, should we say, he draws himself *as* Daladier?). In other words, we could talk about a lifting of the primary repression – albeit a partial one, because in the same session Mr E is able to draw both his "coming apart" *and* Daladier, the man who wants to know nothing about truth.

Both the breaking up of body image and orality disorders were also observed in another patient, Mr U, whose hemineglect, unlike in Mr E's case, persisted as a lasting and serious disability.

Severe hemineglect, holes in the body, oral cravings[5]

Mr U is a lecturer at a provincial university. His focus is multidisciplinary research on the Amerindians. He has come to Paris (where he owns a flat) to get medical advice and care for his left-side hemineglect. When he was 50, Mr U needed surgery to remove a benign brain stem tumour, which was diagnosed as a result of his vertigo. After the operation, Mr U presented a transient left hemiplegia due to a right hemispheric CVA. The consequences of the surgery were rather complicated: Mr U needed a tracheotomy and was kept on artificial respiration for several weeks. He has since suffered from permanent tracheal stenosis and dysphagia. He also presents a complete paralysis of the upper eyelid, and, as a result, his right eye is permanently closed. One year after surgery, although his motor recovery is complete and he should be able to walk by himself, Mr U requires permanent assistance from a caregiver. When moving, he constantly bumps into any obstacles on his left. In the corridor, he walks very close to the right wall; his head faces to the right and the left side of his body is turned backwards. He cannot get dressed on his own, as he does not know which side to put on his clothes. He reads only the right quarter of a text. Alongside these manifestations of left hemineglect, he also presents constructional apraxia and problems with reasoning. In addition to these symptoms, the patient's asomatognosia manifested subsequently, when he was participating in an experimental study. He was shown a video of hand movements and asked to identify those he was himself performing with his left hand.[6] Not only did Mr U fail the task completely, but the experimental procedure brought to light the personification of his left hand. When asked, "Did you ever feel as if your left arm did not belong to you?" or "Do you call it by a name?", Mr U answers: "No, I could have sometimes called it the 'pain in the neck' [*l'emmerdeur*]. And I can't mistake it for the arm of my son, who is a few years younger than me. He is the one closest to me. There could be a fantasy of merging. If I can't be sure that it's mine, I think Antoine should have it back." Familiar places have become double: Mr U gets lost in his own flat, because, as he says, the flat has two entrances, one in rue de la Convention, the other in rue Saint-Jacques (an important street for him, since he studied at the Sorbonne and often returns there to do bibliographical research). The top-ographical impossibility[7] is not a problem for Mr U: rue Saint-Jacques, he explains, is indeed located in 5th *arrondissement*, but it runs as far as the 15th. Thus, according to Mr U, there are two "half-flats": two toilets, two bathrooms, so that he never knows which one is nearest to him. In addition, he mentions hallucinatory phenomena, which in a sense stage the events he hopes will occur. For example, he woke up one night seeing a colleague of his (whom he had planned to call the next day) standing at his bedroom's doorstep. He woke up his wife to tell her, then fell asleep again ("I was tired", he says, without taking any position on the reality of this apparition). Mr U regularly bumps into obstacles on his left; he often falls and cannot go outside on his own, as he is unable to find his way or cross the street. Despite these problems, he is planning to soon return to his job and only complains about problems of reading, due to concomitant eye issues. Such serious difficulties more than a year after the CVA do not spell great promise regarding Mr U's recovery. In response to his complaint about reading, he is then offered speech therapy sessions at his home, with a therapist specialising in right-hemisphere syndrome. Occupational and physical therapy are also provided through our outpa-tient clinic. Mr U attends all these sessions for a year. At the same time, I offer him a weekly appointment to talk to me about his neurological prob-lems. Below is a summary of the notes taken by the practitioners involved in his care. They mostly concern Mr U's ideas regarding his body and his pathology, the kinds of relationships he forms with the different clinicians and the impasses of the various attempts at his rehabilitation.

Mr U's ideas about his body and pathology essentially revolve around the difference between right and left, questions of haste, orality, "holes in the body" and the need to rebuild his "shell".

Hemineglect and orality disorders

With his therapists, Mr U tends to talk about his problems in terms of the loss of the sense of left and right: "I am grabbed by the left side. As if the sense of left has disappeared. I don't know which is right or left anymore." When invited to speak about his neurological problems (in particular his hemineglect), he answers: "It's a minor handicap. The adverse consequences of hemiplegia have become somewhat foreign to me; I am being looked after and so I don't have to suffer from them directly." "It's not worth talking about, it's the grain of sand that messed everything up. . . . I was brought down in full flight." But don't these small details require him to rely on permanent help? Yes, he admits, he needs the young woman who accompanies him everywhere, "because I need reference points" and his wife has chosen a psychomotor therapist for him. Why a psychomotor therapist? This is a proof of love expressed by his wife, who has put all this support in place. What kind of reference points does he need? For example, when getting dressed, the fly on his trousers must face north. Also, he has problems with his balance, his knees go weak and, as a result, he is drawn towards the left side, as if by a magnet. These are the small compulsions due to hemineglect. Are there other compulsions? He eats much too fast, as if the food were going to be taken away from him. "Hemineglect is a kind of nagging worry, so that you do things faster. . . . Sometimes my legs go faster than my body." When talking about his eating habits, Mr U touches his mouth and says: "It's as if I wanted to make the most of what's on my plate. Eating makes me relax. It's a compensatory function, you have to fill yourself up to feel satisfied." Mr U related this haste in eating to a similar haste in speaking: "When I am at the table, I interrupt people, as if I was afraid that they won't let me speak."

> I have a tendency to choke; I cough because of the tracheotomy, and as I cough, I start choking, I feel the food piling up, I feel like I can't say something and I swallow in a hurry in order to say what I want to say. In the same way, when my wife comes home and asks me if I need anything, I need it right away, I don't even let her have a shower and relax, I ask her to do the thing right away.

Another time, Mr U describes his hemineglect as follows: He can easily have a fall, he cannot read and has become a messy and noisy eater. By the way, he adds, he now also makes much more noise with his mouth when speaking.

Given that under normal conditions, the constitution of specular image and the repression of the object are intrinsically related processes, it is not surprising to find that these various inopportune oral manifestations are associated with the breaking up of body image (the legs that move faster than the trunk, the loss of the sense of left and right, etc.).

Holes in the body

On his return from a short holiday, Mr U says that he was sleeping a lot. He needed that "as anyone who's had surgery would. It's an attack against the body, the operation and the openings they made to put in all those tubes. The shell is open." This opening of the shell is clearly seen in the two versions of Mr U's self-portrait. He first draws himself "brought down in full flight" (Figure 6.4a) and comments: "I am falling like a bird that has just been shot." When I point out that he seems to be wearing a cape, he says: "The body is like a small garment that floats around a person's centre, which is his brain." I then ask him to make a more classical drawing of his

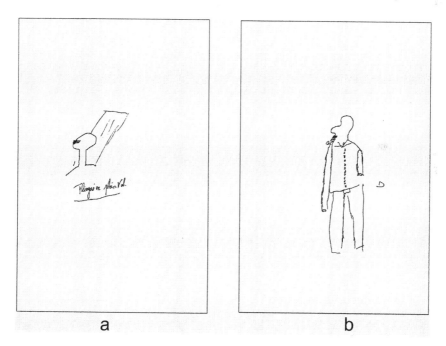

a   b

Figure 6.4 Self-portrait of a right-handed patient with body schema disorders, Mr U
(a) The first version. The patient has written "*Flingué en plein vol*" [brought down in full flight]. (b) The second version, after the patient was asked to draw his body. The letter D written by the patient indicates the right side of the figure. This allows us to see that the portrait is a mirror reflection of the patient.

Source: Morin, C. et al., Qu'est-ce qu'un "gauche" ?, *Annales de Réadaptation et de Médecine Physique*, 2001, 44.

body (Figure 6.4b). He tells me he has drawn a bald head [in French liter-ally "egg-shaped", *en forme decrâne d'oeuf*] and a neck like a stork. "An important head," he says, "that's where it happened." When I ask him to complete his drawing, he does not draw any facial features.

He adds a moustache, saying: "I don't know, I might at least draw my moustache." He talks about the nose (but does not draw it), the ears, the hair ("anyway, there is so little left . . ."). He neither draws nor mentions the mouth, even though it is so present in his discourse. We should note that this portrait shows holes in the body, on the left side of the neck and in the right part of the waist.

The body: a shell that protects the ego

Mr U has certain ideas about the relationships between the body and the self. "I feel my body as a shelter. My family gives me the impression that it's reassuring: I am tall, broad-shouldered. . . . [A]s a child, when I was scolded by a teacher or when I had the kind of fears you can have at school, I would say to myself: 'The self (*moi*) is a shell [*Moi est une carapace*].'" Mr U also says: "When I bump into something because of my hemineglect, my first reaction is irritation: My self escapes me." Mr U feels "irritated" because his illness threatens his entire life project, which consisted in tackling a variety of social issues like Don Quixote – a man hidden in his armour. Although his vexation may at first seem an ordinary narcissistic reaction, it is not unrelated to his visuospatial issues, as shown by the following example. In the same occupation therapy session, this patient declares to his therapist: "Now I'm on bad terms with space, with right and left, and I'm collecting the bits of the mirror together to see if I'm still handsome." His words bring together the functions of body schema and body image: structuring spatial perception and providing an object for narcissism.

Body image disorders also have an effect on the relationships the patient forms with his therapists.

Mr U and his therapists: aggressiveness and transitivism

Aggressive reactions first appeared in the rehabilitation sessions, when the therapists pointed out the problems that Mr U seemed to ignore or deny. His speech therapist felt that her suggestions and advice were experienced as persecutory. Indeed, Mr U includes speech therapy among the things "he would like to get rid of and that are barriers to his autonomy". The list also comprises the need to use eye drops and take medication, MRI scans and the fact that his skin is "dry like parchment paper".

Transitivism characterises many aspects of Mr U's relationships with his therapists, in the sense that the patient tends to assign his own difficulties to others (Wernicke, 1900/2010) and often addresses them in an undifferentiated manner. In one session, his occupational therapist suggests that he draw a map of South America – an area of special interest to him. Due to his left hemineglect, Mr U only draws the states located in the east of the continent. His therapist, who is sitting on his left, then points out this lack to him. Mr U turns leftwards to face her, looks straight into her eyes and exclaims: "Oh but *please*, Danièle, it's *you* who forgot them!", adding transitivism to aggressiveness. In the following session, Mr U comments: "My wife had a good laugh when I told her that you had found my drawing of America *fecalomorphic*."[8] When talking with me, Mr U was never aggressive, which suggests that aggressiveness appeared in response to the therapists' discourse, due to the fact that their job was to identify the pathology behind Mr U's current condition and make him aware of these issues. However, from Mr U's point of view, such statements are aimed at *what he is*, at his *self*, and thus are heard as insults. We can understand that he reacts to them in the paranoid mode. The transitivism that leads him to assign his own errors to his therapist is part of the same tendency, which refers back to a moment close to the mirror stage (Lacan, 1966/2006).

From the very beginning of our sessions, Mr U's position in the dialogue is problematic. At first he says that he is already seeing a psychotherapist and is then told that the idea was for him to talk specifically about the issues for which he is receiving treatment, i.e., his hemineglect. However, as soon as he begins to talk, Mr U leaves his neurological problems completely aside and instead speaks about the changes his illness has caused in his married life. He complains to me and to all his therapists about the regressive aspects of his position (he would like his wife to make a fuss over him the way his mother did; he is afraid of her being angry as he used to be afraid of his father). He never spontaneously speaks of either his hemineglect or his rehabilitation. We meet weekly for a year, while he is also seeing a variety of other practitioners (a haptonomist,[9] an acupuncturist and others). He complains that these sessions are redundant, but does not give up any of them. Most of the time, Mr U seems not to hear any of my comments; however, I am sometimes surprised to hear him report my own words as coming from the acupuncturist. My colleagues notice the same phenomenon – for example, the occupational therapist is allocated the words of the physiotherapist. Mr U reports a dream to his occupational therapist in which his left fingers have been amputated and are running along his right forearm. Although Mr U indicates that he had the dream "after a conversation with Mrs Morin", he never says a word about it to me. Mr U thus addresses the Other in an undifferentiated manner, seemingly regardless of the Other's specific embodiment. This lack of differentiation between his interlocutors can perhaps be put in parallel with an episode of false recognition: Leaving my office after a session, I am walking in front of Mr U, then turn right and disappear from his visual field. At the very same moment, his care assistant (whose clothing and hair are very different from mine) arrives to help him. As she appears right in the spot where I have just disappeared, Mr U tells her: "Goodbye, Dr Morin." All these symptoms – transitivism, aggressiveness, lack of differentiation between others, false recognition – attest to how deeply the patient's subjectivity has been altered by the neurological accident.

Asomatognosia and orality disorders[10]

What we have called *orality disorders* in the cases of Mr E and Mr U may seem rather inconspicuous. As we will see in the following two cases, in other patients these phenomena can manifest in much more spectacular ways. The reports are taken from a study which looked at the discourse of hemiplegic patients in the first seven days after a stroke. Each patient underwent standardised neuropsychological and neurological assessment administered by two different examiners. My role was to carry out semi-directive interviews, during which I was surprised to hear two patients talking about, respectively, biting and kissing. These two patients had suffered cerebral embolism due to heart arrhythmia. Their motor issues, sensory and visual deficiencies, their degree of hemineglect, anosognosia and asomatognosia were assessed in specific sessions.

Mr R: "I saw a left arm passing by and I felt like biting it"

Mr R, age 51, right-handed, is a senior manager suffering from severe left sensorimotor hemiplegia and hemianopsia, together with a visuospatial neglect of both his left hemibody and hemispace. Mr R does his hair on only the left side and with hesitation; in the cancellation test he only crosses out 14 lines out of 40 (the same test that was administered to Mr E, see Figure 1.2). He also exhibits asomatognosia and anosognosia with respect to his left hemiplegia. When asked about a possible movement problem on the left side, he says he feels "no difference at all"; when shown his left hand, he identifies it as belonging to the examiner.

The semi-directive interview shows that the patient's "awareness" of his neurological problems is highly variable. To my surprise, the patient also speaks about an "arm passing by":

CM: Would you like to talk to me about what's happening to you? How are you doing?

Mr R: It could have been worse in terms of distance . . . for example not being able to speak . . .

CM: What has happened to you?

Mr R: I had a stroke . . . no blood was flowing through my brain for a while.

CM: How do you feel?

Mr R: Quite well. Tired, that's normal after an accident . . .

CM: And otherwise?

Mr R: . . .

CM: How's your mood?

Mr R: Things are well taken care of, that's already quite important . . .

CM: Do you think that what happened to you was serious, that your life could have been in danger?

Mr R: Looking back, perhaps the main functions, perhaps not life itself.

CM: The main functions?

Mr R: Sight, speech, the brain capacity . . . but now, after all, the left side, you can retrain that, it's less important than speaking, memory . . .

CM: What's happening with the left side?

Mr R: It doesn't feel like working any more. He is not mistaken, he also worked too much, he wanted to stop, he's like myself.[11]

CM: What do you think about it, about your left side?

Mr R: That with a bit of therapy it will come back, not right away, but still. I ask to get up to go to the toilet.

CM: Do you have dreams at night?

Mr R: I dream that I'm running after the doctors to make them give me a schedule for my future . . . I saw a left arm passing by, I thought it belonged to a caretaker, and I felt like biting it . . .

CM: How do you know that it was a left arm?

Mr R: It was a left arm.

CM: And why this feeling of wanting to bite it?

[Mr R does not answer and remains silent for some time.]

Mr R – Everyone says that I have a left hemiplegia, but I don't feel it. I can move. Everything's possible.

Although Mr R knows he has suffered a cerebrovascular accident, he speaks about his hemiplegia in variable and contradictory terms; he never directly mentions the reality of his deficiency. Moreover, his left arm seems to have a personal life of its own: It has worked too much, like Mr R himself, whom his family describes as 'hyperactive'. When asked about his dreams, Mr R declares: "I saw a left arm passing by and I felt like biting it." He is completely unable to comment on this enigmatic sentence. When I ask why he felt like biting it, he remains silent. He cannot say why he was so certain that it was a left arm. He is not quite sure to whom it belonged. Sometime later his wife tells me that once during this time, Mr R asked her to "pick up something that fell on the floor" – in fact, Mr R's arm had slipped from the arm-rest.

Mr N: "A hand-kissing because I can't shake your hand"

Mr N, age 46, right-handed, is a university professor who previously suffered from hypertension and migraines. He was also a heavy smoker. He presents with a left sensorimotor hemiplegia and a left hemianopsia. He suffers a visuospatial neglect of his left hemispace and hemibody: Mr N does his hair on only the right side and misses 24 lines in the cancellation test. When he is asked "Why are you here?", he first answers: "I've had a cardiovascular accident, I am ill." His asomatognosia is very severe: When shown his own left hand, Mr N identifies it as "your finger" and persists to do so even when I try to make him aware of his error.

In the semi-directive interview, Mr N surprised me a lot when concluding our dialogue with a hand-kissing.

CM: I am working with your doctors to see how people feel after such a serious illness like yours. Would you like to speak with me?

Mr N: I feel very diminished; it's like that with everybody. You [on] feel passive because even the smallest everyday movements are difficult, like grabbing something with both hands.

CM: Why?

Mr N: Because my left hand is paralysed. On Sunday, I had three pains in my head and the next day I realised that I couldn't speak properly, that I had a strange voice and that my leg could not carry me.

CM: How are you feeling?

Mr N: Very tired.

CM: How's your mood?

Mr N: Not great . . . I don't know how long it will take, I've got loads of things to do.

CM: Do you think that what happened to you was serious, that your life could have been in danger?

Mr N: Yes, because these things in the brain, it can get ugly . . . You can become a vegetable . . . You can have a heart attack.

CM: And your left side?

Mr N: I can't feel either my leg or my hand. When I give them an order, nothing happens, I feel as if there is no reflex anymore.

CM: What do you think about your left arm and leg?

Mr N: They are very useful, they are part of myself, it's my body that is mutilated.

CM: If you look at your left hand or touch it, how does it feel?

Mr N: It's as if it was dead, it's not warm, it's cold, it does not have the normal texture of a hand.

CM: Do you dream at night?

Mr N: I dream about the things that are happening in my life. For example, how to organise an association for the prevention of heart disease.

CM: Could you draw a picture of yourself for me?

The patient draws a picture (Figure 6.5).

CM: Is there anything that you would like to add to the picture?

The patient draws a pipe. He adds a double oblong shape above his portrait, which he explains as follows:

Mr N: A kiss because I cannot shake hands . . .
CM: Are there any other things that it would be important to talk about?
Mr N: No.
CM: Well then, I will say goodbye to you.

I extend my hand towards Mr N, who then kisses it.

Mr N: I'm kissing your hand because I cannot shake it.

At first sight, Mr N seems to speak about his paralysed limbs as a neurologist would do: "I can't feel either my leg or my arm", "I feel as if there is no reflex anymore". However, his paralysed hand does provoke a feeling of strangeness. Without any suggestion from myself, Mr N spontaneously wonders whether his limbs belong to his body, yet he answers in the affirmative: "They are part of myself, it is my body that is mutilated." He feels as if his left hand is "dead", since "it does not have the normal texture of a hand" when he touches it. As for the formulation "when I give them an order, nothing happens", it might sound as an expression of the patient's experience of his paralysis. However, the idea of giving an order to the paralysed hand may imply some kind of personification. In addition, hearing Mr N – a right-handed man with left hemiplegia – repeatedly declare that he is unable to shake the other's hand sounds rather peculiar.

The location of the drawing (Figure 6.5) on the right side of the sheet attests to left hemineglect. However, the portrait itself is symmetrical – both hands are represented and occupy most of the space; the trunk is barely present but includes what looks like a heart (located on the right side in the drawing, i.e., like in a mirror image), which corresponds to the patient's concerns regarding his heart disease. Both sides of the lower part of the body are missing, a lack that seems to call for neither an explanation nor a correction. Instead, Mr N spontaneously draws a pipe and smoke. When asked if something might be missing and to complete his drawing, he draws two enormous lips above his portrait and says: "A kiss, because I can't shake hands." Let us note that like Mr R, who in his dreams is chasing

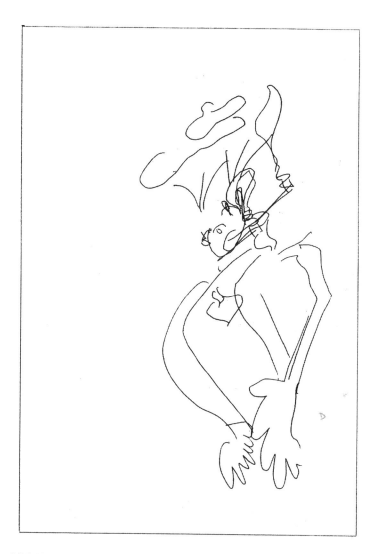

Figure 6.5 Self-portrait of a right-handed patient with body schema disorders, Mr N
The oblong Figure on the left above the portrait's head was drawn secondarily by the patient, who commented: "a hand-kiss, because I can't shake a hand". The letter D written by the patient indicates the right side of the figure. This allows us to see that the portrait is a mirror reflection of the patient.

Source: Morin, C. et al., Asomatognosie et troubles de l'oralité: Une lecture psychanalytique, *Annales de Réadaptation et de Médecine Physique*, 2003, 46.

his doctors to find out something about his future, Mr N also relates his dreams to his current situation, in this case the focus on preventing cardio-vascular disease.

While in the cases of Mr E and Mr R the personification of the hand is relatively muted, in the following cases the symptom is much more foregrounded.

The paralysed hand: a mother's daughter[12]

Mrs M and her daughter-hand with a double leg

Mrs M, aged 67, suffered a right hemispheric CVA due to cardiac arrhythmia. She presents with left hemiplegia, left sensory disorders and left hemianopsia. Mrs M has an asomatognosia: when I show her own left hand to her, she says she sees "a bandage" (which in fact has just been put on her hand) or "nails", which her daughter has painted. When I put her left hand in her right hand, and ask her what it is, she answers: "I don't see what you mean." Because of her anosognosia, she does not complain about her paralysis. Moreover, she says that her grandson has recently accompanied her on a short walk in the hospital garden. The reason why she isn't walking by herself is because she is fastened to her bed and armchair. From the very first days of her illness, Mrs M has been telling her children that her hand was a man's hand and that she [the hand] did not love her any more. She talks to her hand, calls it a naughty girl, she also cajoles it or hits it, or kisses it ("Because I love her all the same"). She hides the hand under her shawl so that it does not catch a cold, so that it can recover. "At night, my hand begins to move, because it's nice and warm under the blanket; during the day, she doesn't want to move, she does the opposite to us: she plays during the night and rests in the daytime – she's lazy. I don't touch her because it's painful. She probably feels abandoned. I tell her I wish she would come back." "In the night, she scratches me, she slips underneath me and scratches me." "She's probably angry with me for not taking good care of her." When asked whom this hand might remind her of, she says she does not want to pronounce the man's name. She then admits that it is in fact her own name, because it belongs to her husband, an alcoholic, who had "more bad sides than good sides" and gave her barely enough money to feed her children. Mrs M then also talks about her childhood, marked by loss and a lack of love, and a question about nomination – abandoned by her mother as a baby, she was only recognised by her father after a legal procedure.

When asked to draw herself (Figure 6.6), she draws her left hand with two legs, wondering aloud: "Why did I draw it with a double leg?"[13] Once she has finished, I ask Mrs M to show me the right and the left hand in the picture. "I can't see the left hand," she answers, "it [*elle*] is

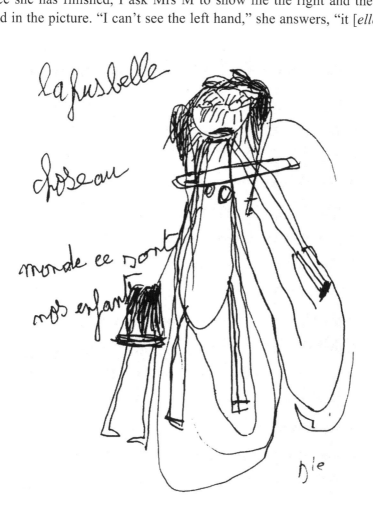

Figure 6.6 Self-portrait of a right-handed patient with body schema disorders, Mrs M
The patient spontaneously wrote: *"Our children are the most beautiful thing in the world."*
The letters Dte written by the patient indicates the right side of the figure. This allows us to see that the portrait is a mirror reflection of the patient.

Source: Morin, Thibierge, Bruguière, Pradat-Diehl, Mazevet, "Daughter-Somatoparaphrenia" in Women with Right-Hemisphere Syndrome: A Psychoanalytic Perspective on Neurological Body Knowledge Disorders, *Neuropsychoanalysis*, 2005, 7.

dead." Mrs M does not draw her mouth. When asked if she would like to add anything, she draws some mascara around her eyes. But it is her daughter who likes to use mascara, while Mrs M never does so. She also adds an extra layer, a coat, she says. Only at my request does she draw her mouth, with the following comment: "A mouth is for speaking, for singing, I don't miss that."

We could say that in this patient, the specular image has been shattered: her hand is not her own, it is "dead" (perhaps we should say that it no longer lives as symbolised in the body image). She speaks of her hand as she would of a difficult child, whom one loves, but who can also be annoying and must be reprimanded. Likewise, her self-image includes traits actually belonging to her daughter. Mrs M also comments that she has drawn her "breasts, which no longer serve any purpose," and then goes on to talk about the love of a mother feeding her children. The comment she spontaneously writes next to her portrait runs along the same lines: "Our children are the most beautiful thing in the world." The multiple circles around the portrait may call to mind the ovum and its membranes, or the idea of swaddling. Most importantly, Mrs M's self-portrait shows us a fragmented body, one that is shared by Mrs M and her daughter.

In addition, this patient again presents with an orality disorder. Not only does she not draw the mouth – as is the case with many elderly people (see Morin and Bensalah, 1998) – but, when this is pointed out to her, her reaction is quite particular. We could argue that the patient's words "I don't miss that" correspond to the formula proposed by Czermak (1986) to account for the distress of patients with Cotard's syndrome: 'the lack of a lack'. Mrs M speaks without pauses or prosodic variations. Her eating habits have changed; she tells us that her children often get cross with her, because she mixes up sweet and savoury foods. Before, she would have never gone out without her braces; now she calmly accepts that because of her facial palsy, they no longer fit. She says that in fact they have never fit her properly, but this would not keep her from eating steak; she is not at all interested in the care team's efforts to arrange a dental appointment. She also suffers from constipation. At first sight, this is a common symptom: what bedridden patients do not complain of constipation? Nevertheless, many patients with left hemiplegia repeatedly insist that they need to pass a stool but cannot. Even at the very beginning of their illness, when the paralysis is most severe, such patients may not complain of their hemiplegia, but instead – as in the above case of Mr R – they protest against not being allowed to get up and go to the toilet.

Mrs M's condition seems to deteriorate. She becomes depressed, refuses to speak and does not recognise me from one meeting to another. Her speech becomes full of negations: "Everything is empty inside. It is as if there were only the bones left, only a carcass." She perceives every act of care as persecutory and rebels against it, often with great determination. She thinks she must be "getting up the nurse's nose": The latter "just keeps repeating [her] name all day long: M . . . M . . . M . . . M . . ." Several months after her stroke and despite daily physiotherapy sessions, Mrs M is still unable to stand up by herself. She does not complain about her hemiplegia, but only about the pains *felt by her left hand:* "She cannot stand the chromed steel of the armchair, it gives her a shock; even me, when I touch her after touching the armchair, it gives her a shock."[14] While saying these words, Mrs M is caressing her hand. When asked what these pains feel like, she keeps caressing it and says: "It burns. It's as if you were choking on something, like something has gone down the wrong way."

The patient's pathology could be understood as a 'body image lesion'. Her hand has a life of its own: it is the hand, rather than Mrs M, that feels pain. It is therefore removed from the body image (Mrs M says "I can't see it, it's dead") and takes on the characteristics of the object. It also shares the object's symbolic relations: it is likened to a child and bears the patient's name. These traits are associated with disorders of the oral realm, with a lack of differentiation in taste (mixing up the flavours) and speech (logorrhoea), as well as with 'Cotard-like' statements. The mouth has lost its symbolic value: Mrs M does not miss it (i.e., does not lack its lack) and says that her paralysed hand suffocates her, as if something had gone down the wrong way.

Mrs C and the daughter left inside her body

Mrs C, age 79, had a right hemispheric stroke due to cardiac arrhythmia. She has long been a widow and had three sons, one of whom died 10 years earlier. Mrs C tells us that when she was six years old, her mother "gave" her to her childless sister, Mrs C's aunt. She presents with left hemiplegia, left sensory disorder and left hemianopsia. Her anosognosia and left hemineglect are very severe and it has been decided that she would be discharged directly into a care home. Nevertheless, Mrs C is planning to organise a large family dinner as soon as she is released from the hospital. Mrs C wonders if she is not losing her head, because she seems to constantly be hearing the voice of her daughter-in-law in the corridor. In her opinion, the woman does not come to the hospital to see her but instead to meet men among the hospital staff. She hears her daughter-in-law repeating the sentence "There is nothing between us" – a phrase that echoes some of Mrs C's own questions. When talking about the key events in her life, she puts great emphasis on a friendship between her and her husband and another couple: "We could have all slept in the same bed, without anything happening." She mentions her hemiplegia only when she complains about the "deadly" smell of her paralysed hand.

When asked to draw herself, Mrs C, whose children are all sons, immediately starts drawing "the daughter we never had" (Figure 6.7). When she eventually agrees to draw herself, she produces a drawing, with perseverations, of a broken-up body, naming the different parts. This body not only lacks its left half (which might be due to left hemineglect), but also its face (Figure 6.7b). Mrs C, whose husband died of Alzheimer's disease, is in fact most of all scared of "losing her head".

Mrs C says that the doctors have arranged for her to see a gynaecologist. She wonders – could they think that she is pregnant? Her perplexity gives some meaning to the formulation "You remained in the cave of my body" [*Tu es restée dans l'antre de mon corps*], which she wrote in a poem addressed to the daughter she never had (Figure 6.7a). In this case, the absence of the left hemibody and the fragmentation of the body image in the self-portrait are accompanied by the "presence" of a daughter neither dead nor alive, who was never given birth to and was left "inside Mrs C's body", together with hallucinatory phenomena around her daughter-in-law, i.e., a different kind of daughter.

Mrs N and her leaf-daughter

Mrs N, a 69-year-old draughtswoman, presents with left sensorimotor hemiplegia and left hemianopsia due to a brain haematoma, a complication of her hypertension. Originally from a Mediterranean country, the patient had a younger brother who died two years earlier and has a younger sister. She is married and childless. She explains that she

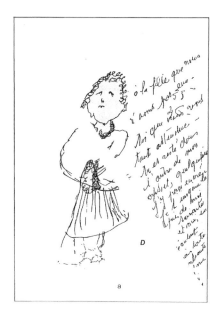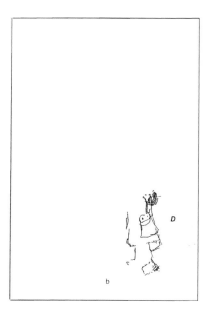

Figure 6.7 Self-portrait of a right-handed patient with body schema disorders, Mrs C, with a poem written by her

(a) A portrait of "the daughter we never had". Note the outline of the arm on the left is partially lacking (left hemineglect).

Source: Morin, Corps, image spéculaire et objet en neurologie, *Bulletin de l'Association Freudienne Internationale*, 1998, 77. Reused by permission of Association Lacanienne freud-lacan.com.

Text of Mrs C's poem:

To the daughter we never had
You, whom we waited for for so long, you remained inside my body.
And sometimes I still think of that. I imagine you, smiling, near me.
And I would be very pleased to hear you, you would tell me "Mummy, don't be afraid, I am here and I will help you do your last steps, as you did when I was a little child and you taught me all the everyday things.

Note the dysgraphia due to left hemineglect.

(b) Mrs C's self-portrait: Mrs C designates "my coat", "my bag", "my hair". The letter D written by the patient indicates the right side of the figure. This allows us to see that the portrait is a mirror reflection of the patient.

Source: Morin, Pradat-Diehl, Robain, Bensalah, Perrigot, Stroke hemiplegia and specular image: lessons from self-portraits, *International Journal of Aging and Human Development*, 2003, 56.

preferred to dedicate herself to creative work; however, she says that this choice was greatly encouraged by her husband, a mathematician, whom she describes as a somewhat rigid personality. She herself – an artist, but no bohemian – divides her time between her solitary walks through Paris and her drawing sessions. In her work, she draws things that attracted her attention on her walks or the landscapes and scenes from her childhood. Mrs N presents with severe hemineglect: She ignores anyone on her left-hand side; every day she is seen wearing her glasses askew, the left earpiece falling across her left ear. She cannot keep looking straight ahead; her gaze is permanently directed below and to the right. Like Mrs C, she spends several months in the rehabilitation department, but still cannot walk on her own. When informed that she will likely not recover much beyond her current state, she becomes greatly reproachful towards her doctor and her physiotherapist ("One can't speak like that to a patient!"), adding, with no apparent emotion, that she will not commit suicide because of her religious convictions. She nevertheless continues to make unrealistic plans (going to a restaurant with a friend, unless he would be embarrassed to be seen with a woman with a cane); she tries to get up by herself and falls. She insists that she has recently managed getting up on her own and followed the doctor to his consulting room. She often smiles, but, combined with her oblique gaze, her "little smile" makes her carers slightly uncomfortable. She tells them she has given her paralysed hand a name, which means "leaf" in her native language, and that she did so because leaves turn green again every year. She also says that she calls her hand her "leaf-daughter" and treats it like the young sister she used to take care of when she was a little girl ("She was my living doll," she says). This daughter has a "symbolic birthday" (the date of the stroke) and her own "cradle" (the arm-rest of Mrs N's wheelchair). Like her younger sister, who, as a teenager, used to borrow Mrs N's clothes, her hand-daughter is very fashion conscious (she requires bracelets and dresses) and somewhat tyrannical (e.g., she demands that people phone and check in on her regularly). She speaks with the same sister's voice. The voice does not have the characteristics of a psychotic voice: It makes relatively ordinary comments on the patient's hospital stay or family life and does not interfere with N's thoughts. The comments are neither offensive nor enigmatic; they bring "consolation" to Mrs N. She herself says that they are not a "hallucination". She does not *really* believe that her hand is a child. It is rather like a kind of scenario, she says, that she has constructed to console herself. When I suggest she draw her arm and hand after she has drawn a picture of herself (Figure 6.8a), she draws an actual arm, not a child (Figure 6.8b). However, she follows the logic of

a   b

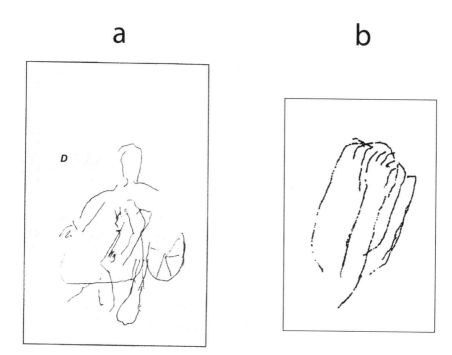

Figure 6.8 Self-portrait of a right-handed patient with body schema disorders, Mrs N
(a) Self-portrait; (b) the hemiplegic arm on the arm-rest of the wheelchair. The letter D
written by the patient indicates the right side of the figure.

Source: Morin, Corps, image spéculaire et objet en neurologie, *Bulletin de l'Association Freudienne
Internationale*, 1998, 77. Reused by permission of Association Lacanienne freud-lacan.com.

her argument all the way: Perhaps her "daughter" will have psychological problems due to her unnatural birth and her very special relationship
to her mother. This daughter will never leave Mrs N, because she will
be buried with her. In addition, without forcing the interpretation, we
might notice that the elements represented on the right-hand side of the
portrait – an arm and two legs – (Figure 6.8a) could seem to figure a kind
of little double inside the portrait.

    In summary, the paralysed arm is associated with a heterogeneous series
of elements (an evergreen leaf, a sister-daughter, a living doll), which are
all connected through the signifier "daughter." For Mrs N, this daughter-
arm-double has a consoling quality.

Mrs S and her daughter-arm stuck in a foetal position

Mrs S, aged 40, was a senior manager of a bank. Divorced, she lives with her three children: a son and two daughters, the youngest nicknamed "Mimi". Throughout her rehabilitation process, her undefeated attitude earns her much sympathy from the staff. She presents with left hemiplegia due to an extended right hemispheric ischemia caused by the rupture of a middle cerebral artery aneurysm. I meet her eight months after her stroke. At the time, she is still unable to walk by herself.

The patient mentions that she experienced 'illusions' six months prior to our meeting, while she was in intensive care. On my request, she later described these illusions in writing. Her short text, written two years after the stroke, presents most of the characteristics of her case with remarkable acuity. It is accompanied by a drawing intended to depict her mental state at the time of her 'illusions' (Figure 6.9). The self-portrait shows evidence of a lasting body schema disorder, which can be attributed to left hemineglect. In her text, there is a marked uncertainty about the ownership of the paralysed arm ("the arm"/"my arm").

This arm is both her own and her daughter's; it still shows traces of paste from adhesive bandages; it is in the "foetal position." Moreover, Mrs S's place of enunciation is ambiguous. Although she claims to be speaking about past illusions, she seems to find it hard to completely detach herself from these thoughts, which once seemed so obvious to her: "The staff refused to believe it and kept saying that it was my arm. I alone knew the truth which, nevertheless, seemed obvious." In French, the formulation "I alone knew" contains a noticeable spelling mistake, the only one in a text written by a highly educated person: Mrs S writes *moi seule savait* instead of *moi seule savais*, using the third person of the verb rather than the first. This ambiguity of the subject with respect to knowledge and truth, which is of great interest to a neurologist interested in psychoanalysis, was already noticeable in our first meeting. The detours and impasses in my conversation with Mrs S clearly show her hesitation and my embarrassment. My lack of understanding and the resulting requests for explanation eventually lead Mrs S to share a highly significant observation:

Mrs S: It was strange for me, because I was telling the truth, but all the doctors told me it was not true. So, I guess that it was perhaps me who did not have my head on straight.

à Mme Morin

Souvenirs d'ailleurs

. le bras
Mon bras gauche était nu et replié (en position fœtale)
il portait des traces blanches comme des marques de
colle laissées par des pansements. en fait c'était le bras
de ma fille Mimi elle avait voulu un câlin près de moi
et nous étions restées soudées. Le personnel ne voulait
pas le croire et soutenait que c'était mon bras. moi seule
savait la vérité qui semblait pourtant évidente

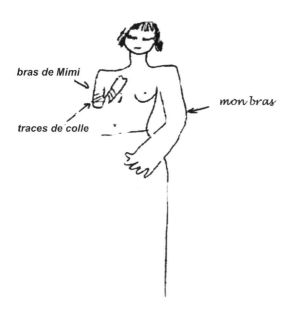

bras de Mimi

mon bras

traces de colle

Figure 6.9 Self-portrait of a right-handed patient with body schema disorders, Mrs S, with
an account of her early illusions, written by her.
"Memories from elsewhere.
My left arm was naked and tucked in (in the foetal position). It had white traces, like paste marks
left by bandages. Indeed, it was my daughter's arm. She had wanted a cuddle with me and we
had remained joined together; the staff refused to believe me and insisted that it was my arm. I
alone knew the truth which, however, seemed obvious."
The arrows indicate "my arm", "Mimi's arm", "traces of paste". The leg on the left is not
drawn due to hemineglect.

CM:	Yes, what did you think of it, then?
Mrs S:	I said that it was not my arm. I said that I was convinced that I had fallen asleep with my daughter in my arms. So, my daughter had put her arm around me. So it was her arm. Yes, and I told everybody that it was not my arm because it was hers. And all the doctors said: No, T, really, it is your arm!
CM:	[. . .] for you, it was her arm? Was it an idea of yours or whenever you looked at it [. . .] you had the impression that it was Mimi's arm?
Mrs S:	No, it was in my head. It was an idea I had.
CM:	When you looked at your arm, what did you see?
Mrs S:	Well, I saw an arm. But between hers and mine [. . .]
CM:	An arm is an arm in some ways . . . but for example, the clothes . . . Had you noticed that it was the same sweater or anything like that?
Mrs S:	No, because I think it was bare.
CM:	It was bare?
Mrs S:	Yes.
CM:	And so, it would have been wrapped around you?
Mrs S:	[putting her left hand on her right shoulder] Yes [. . .]
CM:	Do you know when this disappeared?
Mrs S:	The feelings when I thought it was my daughter? I think it happened because they told me that it wasn't true.
CM:	Because otherwise, you felt like it was true?
Mrs S:	Oh, yes!
CM:	And when, for example, you saw your daughter . . . That arm of hers.
Mrs S:	Oh! I never told her, I didn't . . .
CM:	Well, I understand, but in your mind, if it were there around you, would it mean she had another arm, or how did that work?
Mrs S:	No, it meant that she had held me so tightly in her arms that it had left an imprint . . . to be more precise.
CM:	So you mean, she had kept her arm and you kept the imprint . . .
Mrs S:	And my older daughter told me that during the first week after I came out of the coma, I did not recognise my daughter. I said, "That is not my daughter . . ." Always the same daughter, too, you'd think the other makes less of an impression on me. And I said, "That is not my daughter."

What Mrs S does not say – as if she had forgotten this episode – is what had happened three months after her stroke, when she met a new speech thera-pist. This therapist noted down the encounter in the following terms: "We met for the first session of her therapy, and I was talking to Mrs S to get to know her better and find out about her interests. Talking about her daugh-ters, Mrs S suddenly stopped and wanted to introduce one of her daughters to me. Imagine my surprise, when she caught her left arm, caressed it and began to speak to it: 'Mimi, say good morning, are you here?' After I ques-tioned her a little, she eventually acknowledged her error, but did not seem very upset: OK, her daughter was not here, but having confounded her own limb with her daughter did not seem to disturb her."

There was another remarkable incident. Running into me one morn-ing, Mrs S told me she had just had a very strange feeling. She felt that something was wrong, that she had forgotten something, and suddenly she realised what it was: she had "forgotten her left arm at home". She added: "I was afraid I would be told off by my physiotherapist!" Mrs S told me about this experience as something rather odd, but she did not make any judgement about the real possibility of a person forgetting her arm.

As in the previous cases, Mrs S's case associates a fragmentation of body image with the incongruous presence of a figure/object that inter-feres with this image.

Notes

1 The findings of this research were previously published in Morin, Thibierge and Perrigot (2001).

2 This performance suggests that the patient is able to shift his attention leftwards, but only to an object that strongly interests his psychic life – in this case a fish (a trout), a classic phallic symbol (Freud, 1916). It is as if the object had to be actually present to "animate" the patient.

3 [In French, the patient says he is *tout déglindé*, i.e., he uses a neologism, a distortion of *tout déglingué:* "wrecked", "falling to pieces", "broken" – Translator's Note.]

4 This syndrome associates anxiety, ideas of being damned or possessed, suicidal ten-dencies, self-mutilation and analgesia with hypochondriac ideas: The organs, the whole body or the world or God are destroyed or no longer exist, and the patient will never be able to die. Czermak (1986) has proposed to interpret these symptoms psy-choanalytically, particularly the negation of organs (especially the orifices). According to his reading, these negations in fact *affirm* a type of completeness – the "lack of a lack" of the object – and are logically associated with the failure of the specular image. Such patients, who often claim that they have no mouth anymore, have no specular image ("I am scattered in space, like objects") and no longer perceive the world

("I have no brain anymore, I don't think anymore, my brain is congested"). This symptomatic structure common to both psychosis and RBI could open a way to an understanding of the occurrence of psychotic-like manifestations following RBI (Ellis, 1994).

5 The findings of this research were previously published in Morin, Taillefer et al. (2001).

6 The patient's hand is covered in a yellow glove; at the same time he is shown a video of a moving yellow hand. Some movements are those he is performing himself, shown in real time. Others are 'fake' movements performed by another person. The patient must identify which movements are his own (see Sirigu, Daprati, Pradat-Diehl, Franck and Jeannerod, 1999).

7 [Rue de la Convention is located in the 15th *arrondissement* of Paris, while rue Saint-Jacques runs through the 5th *arrondissement* along the Sorbonne – Translator's Note.]

8 The meaning of the patient's neologism is clear enough.

9 Haptonomy is a therapeutic technique focusing on touch in affective relationships.

10 The findings of this research were previously published in Morin, Durand et al. (2003).

11 [We have decided to translate the French *il,* perfectly grammatically appropriate to talk about the patient's arm [*le bras*] as "he", to underline the personification of this body part – Translator's Note.]

12 The findings of this research were previously published in Morin (1998), Morin et al. (2003), Morin, Thibierge, Bruguière, Pradat-Diehl and Mazevet (2005).

13 The personification of the hand reminds us the Preyer's observation, quoted in Wallon (1931) in the latter's study of the development of the notion of one's own body in children: "Although they are recognized and individualized, the child does not immediately integrate his body parts in his physical individuality. Aged 1 year and 11 months, the child [in Preyer's observation] repetitively offers a biscuit to his own foot, as he does to his parents, and greatly enjoys the toes being able to catch it [our translation]." Scupin (also quoted by Wallon) reported that another child put his naked calves on the balcony "so that they can see the world", just like he moved stones in the garden to "make them see something new".

14 [Again, we translate the French *elle,* appropriate to talk about the patient's hand [*la main*] as "she", to underline the personification of this body part – Translator's Note.]

References

Czermak, M. (1986). Signification psychanalytique du syndrome de Cotard. In J. Clims (Ed.), *Passions de l'objet* (pp. 205–236). Paris: Editions de l'Association Freudienne.

Ellis, H.D. (1994). The role of the right hemisphere in the Capgras delusion. *Psychopathology, 27,* 177–185.

Freud, S. (1916). Symbolism in dreams. *Standard edition, 15,* 149–169.

Freud, S. (1925). Negation. *Standard Edition, 19,* 235–239.

Joanette, Y., Goulet, P., Hannequin, D. (1990). *Right hemisphere and verbal communication.* New York: Springer Verlag.

Lacan, J. (2006). The mirror stage as formative of the I function as revealed in psychoanalytic experience. In *Ecrits* (pp. 75–81). New York: Norton. (Originally published 1966)

Morin, C. (1998). Corps, image spéculaire et objet en neurologie. *Bulletin de l'Association Freudienne Internationale*, *77*, 7–11.

Morin, C., Bensalah, Y. (1998). Self-portrait in adulthood and aging. *International Journal of Human Aging and Development*, *46*, 45–70.

Morin, C., Durand, E., Marchal, F., Timsit, S., Manai, R., Pradat-Diehl, P., Rancurel, G. (2003). Asomatognosie et troubles de l'oralité: Une lecture psychanalytique. *Annales de Réadaptation et de Médecine Physique*, *46*, 12–23.

Morin, C., Pradat-Diehl, P., Mazevet, D., Gautherin, D., Weill-Chounlamountry, A., Dubail, M., Robain, G. (2003). Un enfant dans le bras. Un trouble féminin de l'image du corps en neurologie? *Bulletin de l'Association Lacanienne Internationale*, *101*, 13–22.

Morin, C., Taillefer, C., Vallat, C., Helsly, N., Thibierge, S., Pradat-Diehl, P. (2001). Qu'est-ce qu'un "gauche"? *Annales de Réadaptation et de Médecine Physique*, *44*, 192–204.

Morin, C., Thibierge, S., Bruguière, P., Pradat-Diehl, P., Mazevet, D. (2005). "Daughter-somatoparaphrenia" in women with right hemisphere syndrome: A psychoanalytical perspective on neurological body knowledge disorders. *Neuropsychoanalysis*, *7*, 47–60.

Morin, C., Thibierge, S., Perrigot, M. (2001). Right brain damage, body image and language: A psychoanalytic perspective. *Journal of Mind and Behavior*, *22*, 69–89.

Sirigu, A., Daprati, E., Pradat-Diehl, P., Franck, N., Jeannerod, M. (1999). Perception of self-generated movement following left parietal lesion. *Brain*, *122*, 1867–1874.

Wallon, H. (1931). Comment se développe la notion du corps propre chez l'enfant. *Journal de Psychologie*, *28*, 705–748.

Wernicke, C. (2010). *Grundriss der Psychiatrie in klinischen Vorlesungen*. Whitefish, MT: Kessinger Publishing. (Originally published 1900)

Chapter 7

Right-hemisphere syndrome: physiopathological hypotheses

The cases presented in Chapter 6 display most of the aspects of what neurologists call right-hemisphere syndrome, or RHS (Carota, Annonia, Piccardi and Bogousslavsky, 2005). In everyday life, patients with RHS can walk around the rehabilitation service half-shaved or with half of their face made up; they can be dressed incorrectly (for example, with their left trouser leg half down). They can confuse their caregivers and might not be able to find their room; despite their paralysis, they might try getting up and they fall. In these patients, cognitive disorders are associated with body schema disorders. In their review of these disorders, Carota et al. (2005) note "a reduced sensitivity to new information, emotional content and non-verbal, gestural information", "a tendency to intrusion and confabulation, a poor understanding of the other's intentions, of the temporalities of a conversation, of metaphors, analogies and proverbs". However, this list fails to show us the specificities of *being* a patient with a right brain injury (Morin, 2006). Indeed, among neurologists – who traditionally have little interest in subjective considerations – RHS seems to provoke some rather surprising comments. In his report to a French-speaking Conference on Psychiatry and Neurology, Barbizet (1972) described "the fate of the patient with permanent left hemiplegia" as follows: "He can only survive by undergoing a deep regression and is lucky if some maternal hands and voice decide to take care of him." Barbizet notes a "real disembodiment of language" in these patients. During the same conference, Delahousse (1972) ventured to propose a psychoanalytic reading of "the anosognosic attitude of left hemiplegic patients". In his view, in some patients the paralysed arm can be given the status of the object in the psychoanalytic sense of the term. Laplane's list of "strange phenomena" in neurology (1998) includes the "deliriums" of right-hemisphere patients concerning their paralysed hand. More recently, Carota et al. (2005) conclude their didactic chapter of the *Encyclopédie médico-chirurgicale* by describing their 'impression' of right-hemisphere patients. On the one hand, they offer a cognitivist interpretation of the role of the right hemisphere, which would be part of a "multi-modal and diffuse network involved in self-consciousness"; on the other hand, they "feel" that patients with right-hemisphere lesions are "less alive, less connected individuals". In other words, neurology has not been able to fully account for the behaviour of RBI patients in terms of well-defined symptoms. It can identify asomatognosia, anosognosia, hemineglect and somatoparaphrenia; it may note, following Jean Lhermitte (1939/1998), that these disorders affect self-consciousness. And yet there is something about how right-hemisphere patients behave, a kind of "je-ne-sais-quoi", which calls for epithets such as "strange" or "disembodied". The difficulties of neurologists can be contrasted with the habitual certainty shown by rehabilitation teams, who will often respond to certain peculiarities in the discourse or behaviour of RBI patients by "S/he is a leftie [*C'est un gauche*]." This implies that RBI patients present with, on the one hand, body schema disorders and, on the other hand, a specific way of being that an experienced therapist can identify but cannot explain or express any better than a neurologist. Before offering a psychoanalytic interpretation of this fact, I will first look at how the question has been treated in recent literature.

Cognitivist hypotheses

Some authors claim that the changes to body schema due to a right-brain lesion can "provoke" somatoparaphrenia as a reaction to the deficiencies in perceiving or integrating body-related information. Gandola et al. (2011) suggest that the "left hemispheric narrator" is deprived of the information normally received from the right hemisphere and might therefore construct aberrant rationalizations. A similar interpretation is offered to explain the delusions of influence in schizophrenic patients. Such patients present with the delusion that their thoughts and gestures are imposed on them by an external and persecutory agent; some authors consider that the basis of this disorder is a "false attribution" of the origin of their acts (Jeannerod, 2003).[1] This line of reasoning cannot but raise the following question: From what perspective are such parallels between neurological and psychiatric syndromes justified? Based on a comparison between the discourse and symptoms of Fregoli and somatoparaphrenic patients, in our previous work we have in fact also put forward a physiopathological hypothesis (Morin and Thibierge, 2006). However, this does not necessarily imply that both disorders employ the same mechanism. Plus, we must ask whether it is legitimate to equate the brain lesions caused by a stroke with the variations in brain metabolism observable via functional MRI. First we must keep in mind that following a limb injury any normal subject can have strange feelings, without these developing into a somatoparaphrenia or a paranoiac delusion. For example, Michaux (1994) describes his sensations after a fracture of the olecranon process, complicated by an algodystrophy: "Since this morning, to my right, to my right which is no longer an arm, which is no longer embers, a piece of furniture" (p. 246). Michaux's words might sound like somatoparaphrenia, if he did not add, a few paragraphs later: "I look ten, twenty times. Looking exists to correct one's impressions" (ibid). In other words, Michaux questions his feelings and thoughts. Brain injured patients devoid of RHS do the same: When they have sensory disorders, they say things like: "It's *as if* my hand did not belong to me." This is completely different from the words of psychotic patients, who are *convinced* that a malevolent force has taken control of their bodies; in fact, they sometimes actively try to defend themselves. It is also different from the discourse of somatoparaphrenic patients, who simply *affirm* that their hand belongs to somebody else. More generally, terms such as *delirium*, *delusion* and *hallucination*, which are sometimes used to describe the symptomatic production of RHS, are essentially part of psychiatric symptomatology. In this field, they qualify thoughts or discourse that diverge from what is generally accepted as reality. However, classical French psychiatry has long made a distinction between delusional discourse – which sounds artificial or incomprehensible and interferes with the patient's thought (Ey, 1948, p. 245) – and so-called *oniroïd* disorders, where "affective projections" are easily identified (Ey, 1948, p. 361). In fact, the somatoparaphrenic themes are not just any themes; as Feinberg (2010) also notices, they are not free of "affective projections". This is clear in certain cases of 'rationalizations', such as those reported by Gandola et al. (2011). A male patient wonders about the gender of his hand's owner

("It's not a man's hand"). A female patient attributes her hand to "that handsome doctor". Such personal, affective and sexual connotations are also found in our patients' discourse. To better illustrate the difference between psychosis and somatoparaphrenia, let us compare the cases of Mrs C, who thought she might be pregnant at the age of 79, and the observation of a psychotic patient reported by Czermak (1998). Although Czermak's patient was in her sixties and post hysterectomy, she had an unwavering conviction that she would give birth to twins, fathered by a well-known public figure. While this patient did not seem at all perplexed as to the feasibility of such pregnancy, Mrs C is quite astonished and laughs at the idea – she says that her doctors "perhaps think" that she is pregnant. Likewise, although she is convinced that all day long she has been hearing her daughter-in-law pronouncing the words "there is nothing between us" behind her room's wall, she wonders whether this might mean that she is going mad. Above all, her 'hallucination' of a depraved daughter-in-law echoes her own life story and her questions about what 'there is' or 'isn't' between men and women. Similarly, the poem she dedicates to the daughter she never had (Figure 6.7) is an appeal made in her present state of helplessness ("You would say: Mummy, don't be afraid, I'm here and I'll always help you do your last steps"), at a moment when all her sons and daughters-in-law have decided, following medical advice, to put her in a retirement home. In the two other cases of "daughter-somatoparaphrenia", the odd premise that a child is present in or as the patient's own arm also follows a neurotic logic. Mrs S wonders about what each of her two daughters means to her ("As if the older daughter made less of an impression on me"). Mrs N comments on the problems caused by an excessively close mother-daughter relationship and on the possibility of separation ("She [the hand] will never leave me, because she will follow me to the grave"). Still, such speculations can often sound stereotyped, as if inspired by a received wisdom rather than a personal concern. Indeed, during her many psychotherapy sessions with the clinical psychologist in the department, Mrs S never spontaneously brought up her strange ideas about her paralysed hand, nor did she allude to them possibly being connected to her close relationship with her daughters or the conflicts that repeatedly arose between her and other women in the family.

To conclude, hemiplegic patients with neurological disorders of body image present us with a specific discourse, the tone of which differs from both the discourse of other hemiplegic patients and the delusions of paranoia.

Right-hemisphere syndrome, image and object

The question we have so far not touched on is, how can the presence of a brain lesion lead to a given type of delusional discourse? From the words and drawings of both normal subjects and hemiplegic patients devoid of RHS we know that metaphorical language invests the hands with high symbolic and imaginary value (phallus-hand). These associations must have brain inscriptions, which right-brain lesions might interrupt, thus revealing the hand's object-status. More generally, we could argue that the relationship between image and object provides a heuristic template to describe what happens when, due to an alteration in our neuronal circuitry, our specular "construction" fails to structure our world. From everyday psychopathology we already know that a simple wavering of our specular image produces an experience of what Freud has called the "uncanny" (1919). And as Lacan shows in his seminar on anxiety (2004/2014), this strangeness, this loss of what is familiar, what is "home" – in other words, our transitory inability to match our thoughts to our body image – has something to do with the intrusion of the object. As discussed in the previous chapter, it is precisely the object's abrupt emergence that manifests, in different forms, in the speech of RHS patients. At times this may be an oral object (the passing arm Mr R wants to bite into or Mr N's unexpected hand-kissing). Another man, whom I met several years after his stroke, was somewhat surprised when he remembered that he and his fellow patient used to have a kind of running joke between them, pretending that the hospital food was made of patients' corpses. The concerns with defecation, which are often seen as self-evident and not given sufficient consideration, are in fact expressed almost exclusively by RHS patients (Morin, 2006). RHS patients may also treat their paralysed hand as a relative, often one whose status as an object for the patient is paramount. This clearly appears in female patients who treat their paralysed hand as a child. In fact, in female psychic life a child often represents the phallic object (Freud, 1933). Something similar can be heard in the words of a male patient, Mr L, who treated his hand as a woman of loose morals. He called his hand *"ma cocotte"*,[2] adding: "She really could do something for me, the bitch! [*Elle pourrait bien faire quelque chose pour moi, la sal . . . !*]." I asked him: "*Ma cocotte . . .* is there somebody who you call *ma cocotte*, perhaps your wife?" "Oh no!" Mr L exclaimed, shocked: "I would never dare! My wife, I call her honey [*ma biche*]."[3] Here we see the classical split in the masculine attitude towards women (Freud, 1912), who are either idealised (the mother) or reduced to a sexual object (the prostitute). Mr L equates his hand with the latter. The paralysed arm is thus given the status of the object. Lacan (1953) reports a similar example, with the dream of a patient born with a brachial plexus palsy. After beginning his medical studies, the patient reports a dream in which his rectum appears in his axilla, i.e., near the place that contains his injured brachial plexus.[4]

We have already discussed the semiological differences between somatoparaphrenia and psychosis. However, it is important to stress that both pathologies combine, albeit in very different forms, a fragmentation of body image and the presence of the object in the patient's psychic life. In psychotic patients, the lost object, which re-emerges in the discourse of RHS patients, has in fact never been lost; instead, according to an adage attributed to Lacan, the patients carry it "in their pocket". It would of course be unreasonable to look for some common organic cause[5] purely on the basis of this analogy. However, the parallel does imply that certain structural elements of the psyche are shared by all speaking subjects, healthy or ill. Specifically, the study of the different modes of body image disorders strongly suggests that the relationship between a stable specular image and a psychically present object is one of mutual exclusion.

As argued by Thibierge (2011), the dismantling of the specular image has effects on our ability to perceive and recognise reality. We cannot simultaneously identify the object and recognise our world (our 'reality') as familiar. The example of Mrs S is highly instructive: she did not recognise her daughter as part of reality ("That's not my daughter"), instead identifying her as the "excessively present" object (the embodiment of a child, a piece of the patient's body that was never lost). That the stability of the image is never compatible with the presence of the object, regardless of the pathology in question, suggests that this mutual exclusion is inscribed in the architecture of the brain over the course of individual development. The discourse of neurological patients thus brings to light the bodily antecedents of the object, which orient our desire and our relationships with others. From this perspective, RHS is of interest to psychoanalysts for more than one reason. On the one hand, it reveals what is ordinarily hidden and needs analysis and interpretation to take shape (Thibierge and Morin, 2010). On the other hand, if the RHS syndrome basically consists of a disturbance of the patient's relationship to his object, the question of how an RBI patient can mourn the motor or cognitive functions altered by a stroke merits a psychoanalytic reading.

Such a reading may help neurologists revisit some of the discussions on the nature of anosognosia, insofar as psychoanalysis considers that our *gnosia* – i.e., our knowledge and recognition of reality – is structured by our body image. If this image happens to be distorted, what we consider 'reality' may change. The attitude of patients with somatoparaphrenia or hemineglect illustrates this hypothesis very well. Somatoparaphrenia provokes a feeling of strangeness in others, but not in the patient himself. Mrs S (see above) is thus able to say "I alone knew the truth", when she describes what she nevertheless calls her 'illusions'. Likewise, patients with hemineglect who fail to see an object situated on their left may not seem either astonished or relieved when somebody points it to them. It feels like the left hemispace is simply not part of their world, as if they had a 'new body image', one that will from now on 'format' their reality in a different way. In the next two chapters, we will first consider the implications of psychoanalytic reflections on anosognosia. The problem of mourning and acceptance of hemiplegia in patients presenting with RHS will also be discussed. These questions are interrelated, because for Freud, mourning is a movement from a neurotic *méconnaissance* of a loss towards gradually becoming aware of the series of significant traits of what has been lost. However, becoming aware of their impairment – in other words, of the particular traits of the loss caused by stroke – is precisely the process that anosognosic patients seem unable to complete.

Notes

1 We should remember that Séglas (1892) already showed that verbal hallucinations can correspond to the words produced by the patient himself.

2 [While *ma cocotte* is a term of endearment, *une cocotte* can designate a woman of loose morals – Translator's Note.]

3 [In French, literally "my little doe" – Translator's Note.]

4 One could ask whether the paralysed arm or hand is thought of in terms of the object precisely because it is lost, as the object inherently is? Or is it because of the special metaphorical value of the left hand (the "bad" hand for both right-handers and left-handers)? This is a difficult question. It seems that legs and feet are not personified in

the same way, not even in patients in whom the hemiplegia mostly affects the lower limbs. Yet, this argument does not hold, because in such cases the cerebral lesions are located elsewhere and do not affect body schema.

5 A neurologist might be tempted to assign a right hemispheric location to body image. However, in my experience, most of the spectacular cases of body image disorders are observed in patients with widespread or multiple brain lesions, i.e., lesions which may disconnect the right hemisphere from other parts of the brain. It seems therefore reasonable to say, quite in agreement with both the hypothesis of Jean Lhermitte (1939/1998) and modern data (Melzack, 1990; Vogeley and Fink, 2003), that crucial knots in the neuronal circuitry responsible for body schema and body image – rather than a supposed "body image centre" – are located in the right hemisphere.

References

Barbizet, J. (1972). Le monde de l'hémiplégique gauche: essai de théorisation. In *Compte Rendu du 70ᵉ Congrès de Psychiatrie et de Neurologie de Langue Française* (pp. 1033–1054). Paris: Masson.

Carota, A., Annonia, J.M., Piccardi, L., Bogousslavsky, J. (2005). Syndromes majeurs de l'hémisphère mineur. *Encyclopédie médico-chirurgicale, Neurologie, 2*, 475–504.

Czermak, M. (1998). On m'arlequine la mentalité. Du caractère irrésistible et traumatique du transfert dans les psychoses. In J. Bergès (Ed.), *Patronymies. Considérations cliniques sur les psychoses* (pp. 96–101). Paris: Masson.

Delahousse, J. (1972). Considérations sur l'attitude anosognosique de l'hémiplégique gauche. In *Actes du 70ᵉ Congrès de Psychiatrie et de Neurologie* (pp. 1082–1088). Paris: Masson.

Ey, H. (1948). Structure des psychoses aiguës et déstructuration de la conscience. In *Etudes psychiatriques, vol 3*. Paris: Desclée de Brouwer.

Feinberg, T.E. (2010). Neuropathologies of the self: A general theory. *Neuropsychoanalysis, 12*, 133–158.

Freud, S. (1912). On the universal tendency to debasement in the sphere of love. *Standard Edition, 11*, 177–190.

Freud, S. (1919). The uncanny. *Standard Edition, 17*, 219–256.

Freud, S. (1933). Anxiety and instinctual life. *Standard Edition, 22*, 81–101.

Gandola, M., Invernizzi, P., Sedda, A., Ferrè, E.R., Sterzi, R., Sberna, M., Paulesu, E., Bottini, G. (2011). An anatomical account of somatoparaphrenia. *Cortex, 48*, 1165–1178.

Jeannerod, M. (2003). The mechanism of self recognition in humans. *Behavioural Brain Research, 142*, 1–15.

Lacan, J. (1953). Some reflections on the ego. *International Journal of Psychoanalysis, 34*, 11–17.

Lacan, J. (2014). *Anxiety: The Seminar of Jacques Lacan, Book X*. Cambridge: Polity Press. (Originally published 2004)

Laplane, D. (1998). L'étrange en neurologie. *Etudes Psychothérapiques, 17*, 23–32.

Lhermitte, J. (1998). *L'image de notre corps*. Paris: L'Harmattan. (Originally published 1939)

Melzack, R. (1990). Phantom limbs and the concept of a neuromatrix. *Trends in Neuroscience, 13*, 88–92.

Michaux, H. (1994). *Darkness Moves: An Henri Michaux Anthology, 1927–1984*. Berkeley and Los Angeles: University of California Press.

Morin, C. (2006). Comportement et lésions hémisphériques droites. In P. Azouvi, J.M., Mazaux and P. Pradat-Diehl (Eds.), *Comportement et lésions cérébrales. Actes des 19es Entretiens de la fondation Garches* (pp. 102–114). Paris: Frison Roche.

Morin, C., Thibierge, S. (2006). Body image in neurology and psychoanalysis: History and new developments. *Journal of Mind and Behavior*, 27, 301–318.

Ramachandran, V.S., Blakeslee, S. (1998). *Phantoms in the Brain. Probing the Mysteries of the Human Mind*. New York: William Morrow.

Séglas, J. (1892). *Des troubles du langage chez les aliénés*. Paris: Rueff et Cie.

Thibierge, S. (2011). *Le nom, l'image, l'objet. Image du corps et reconnaissance*. Paris: Presses Universitaires de France.

Thibierge, S., Morin, C. (2010). The self and the subject a psychoanalytical perspective. *Neuropsychoanalysis*, 7, 81–93.

Vogeley, K., Fink, G.R. (2003). Neural correlates of the first person perspective. *Trends in Cognitive Sciences*, 7, 38–42.

Weinstein, E.A., Kahn, R.L. (1955). *Denial of illness*. Springfield: C.C. Thomas.

Chapter 8

Anosognosia

Anosognosia for hemiplegia is a spectacular phenomenon: A hemiplegic patient seems unaware of what is perfectly visible and obvious, i.e., his inability to move one of his arms or legs. This symptom has been described at length in neurological literature (see Ellis and Small, 1993; Vocat, 2010). In hemiplegic patients, anosognosia mostly concerns left hemiplegia, due to a left-hemispheric brain lesion. The causal lesions are often widespread and may affect several zones of the right frontal, temporal, and parietal lobes. The most commonly affected are the dorsal premotor cortex, the inferior parietal lobule and the insula. In hemiplegics, anosognosia is nearly always associated with negative body schema disorders (left hemiasomatognosia or hemineglect) and sometimes also with a strange discourse regarding the paralysed hemibody: the patients may question the ownership of their paralysed limbs. A variety of physical manoeuvres – for example, vestibular stimulation by injecting cold water into the left ear – may cause both anosognosia and left hemineglect to momentarily disappear (Cappa, Sterzi, Vallar and Bisiach, 1987). In addition, many other aspects of anosognosia are revealed in the day-to-day care for patients in a rehabilitation department.

Anosognosia in everyday life

Anosognosia may pervade a patient's entire attitude towards his illness. The complete ignorance of hemiplegia usually disappears after several weeks. However, the patient can retain a tendency to minimise his difficulties, to elude any concerns about his future and downplay or dismiss the precautionary rules or rehabilitation principles. Some patients denigrate the boring exercises they are asked to do, instead imagining a kind of "switch" that would suddenly allow them to move as they did before the stroke (Morin,

Thibierge and Perrigot, 2001). Anosognosia concerns not just the current perception of motor deficiency, but the patient's entire range of representations of hemiplegia, present and past. This appears in the way patients typically report on the onset of their hemiplegia: "I fell and I couldn't get up." When asked why they could not get up, they say that they did not know – *and still do not know*. Even after several months in rehabilitation they will not say, "Now I understand that it was because my left leg was paralysed." In the same patient, anosognosia may vary from one moment to another. This is apparent in the dialogue with Mr R (see Chapter 6). During the same interview, Mr R said: "The left side, it could be retrained, it's not so important as speech or memory"; later he added: "With a bit of exercise, it will recover, not immediately, but still"; finally saying: "Everybody tells me I have left hemiplegia. I don't feel it. I can move. Everything is possible" (Morin, Durand et al., 2003). Anosognosic patients often resist when their therapists try to make them aware of their deficiencies and the risks these could entail. The therapist is often surprised by the aggressive reaction of a patient, who may feel mistreated or infantilised.

Cognitive theories of anosognosia

Several cognitive theories have tried to account for anosognosia (see Vocat, 2010; Ellis and Small, 1993). Some authors consider anosognosia as an alteration in the patient's emotional reaction to hemiplegia, due to the asymmetrical distribution of the control over emotions between the two hemispheres. However, most authors interpret anosognosia in terms of some issue in the brain's treatment of external data: either a problem of sensory feedback, which normally confirms that a planned movement has actually been performed, or a difficulty in "detecting" the motor deficiency, or a more general problem in identifying anomalies. Some of these theories rely on the premise of an interhemispheric disconnection (Geschwind, 1965), a general intellectual weakening or an attention disorder. In the end, none of these cognitive theories are able to explain the variability of anosognosia in the same patient. Moreover, they do not take into account the associated disorders of body representation.

Psychological theories of anosognosia

A number of purely psychological theories have also been proposed, identifying anosognosia as a defensive reaction, a form of denial or repression.

The first of these conceptions was presented by Babinski (1914) at the Société de Neurologie in Paris. The famous French neurologist wondered whether the persisting anosognosia in one of his female patients might not be a form of "coquetry", the patient refusing to see herself as disabled.

Anosognosia: a defence against a change in self-image?

Weinstein, a psychiatrist who treated many neurological patients, also considered anosognosia as a means of protecting the patient's own self-image. He used the term *denial,*[1] nevertheless his theorisation evokes normal neurotic *méconnaissance.* In *Denial of Illness* (Weinstein and Kahn, 1955), Weinstein writes: "The effect of the brain damage is to provide the milieu of function in which *any* incapacity or defect may be denied, whether it is hemiplegia, the fact of an operation or an unfortunate life situation" (1955, p. 96; our emphasis). He also writes: "If we use the concept of body scheme, it cannot be 'localised' to any part of the brain as an anatomical representation. It must include not only the physical appearance of the body, but also other spatial, temporal and interpersonal aspects of the relation of the self in the environment. Further, it must include the role of motivation of the individual to preserve his integrity" (p. 37). Most neurologists reject such interpretation, because anosognosia is mostly observed in patients with right-hemisphere lesions (for contrary examples, see Ellis and Small, 1993), which are not prone to undermine the individual's integrity and control any more than left lesions (see e.g., Adair and Barrett, 2011, p. 202). However, the fact that a symptom has an organic basis does not rule out its having a psychological significance as well. Also, understanding the psychic logic of anosognosia might help us in making decisions on how to best rehabilitate anosognosic patients.

Anosognosia: a méconnaissance systématique?

The analogy between anosognosia and *méconnaissance systématique* (Dissez, 2009) has never been examined. However, *méconnaissance systématique*, a severe form of ignorance of major life events, is a spectacular form of rejecting reality. A doctoral thesis by Borel (1931), devoted to the *méconnaissance* of death, discusses cases of psychotic patients living for extended periods of time alongside the corpse of a loved one. Czermak (1998) also uses the term *méconnaissance systématique* when reporting on a female patient who is convinced, despite having undergone hysterectomy, that one day she will give birth to twins. It is true that some anosognosic patients may ignore their paralysis to the point of suffering a fall. However, this happens only episodically and the patients later admit they were careless. I have met only one patient who refused the diagnosis of stroke, challenged the resident physician to prove he really had a stroke and left the emergency unit despite left hemiparesis. Later on, the follow-up and family reports made a strong case for the diagnosis of paranoia.

Anosognosia: a denial?

In this understanding of anosognosia, denial (see note 1) refers to what Freud calls *Verleugnung*, i.e., a process that permits a subject to both admit and refuse castration (Freud, 1938). Delahousse (1972) considers the personification of the paralysed hand a kind of denial, which gives actual presence to the lost object. He reports on a case of a female patient who personified her paralysed hand as her beloved son, who in reality was working abroad. Delahousse thus establishes a relationship between denial and anosognosia as a belief of maintaining control over the paralysed arm. This would mean that the brain lesion allows the lost object to come to the fore, taking on the very form it assumes in the subject's present-day desire or demand. The patient would treat his paralysed arm as a fetish. However, in fetishism, the subject chooses a "fake", stereotyped object, one that has no direct relationship to his current concerns. On the contrary, in RHS patients the object of the demand manifests itself directly, e.g., as the far-away son of Delahousse's patient, the passing arm that can be bitten or the favourite daughter in our own observations.

Anosognosia: a repression?

Ramachandran (Ramachandran and Blakeslee, 1998) claims that anosognosia represents a caricatural form of repression. He bases this assumption on the following observation. He injected cold water in the ear of a patient who had previously denied that she was hemiplegic. Immediately after the injection, the patient admits, when questioned, that she is indeed hemiplegic and has been so for several days. The next morning, she remembers that cold water was put in her ear but does not remember having spoken about her hemiplegia with Dr Ramachandran. Ramachandran sees the episode as an exemplary case of "repression", which he nevertheless understands as intentional forgetting – a rather simplistic conception. The patient's behaviour indicates that the anosognosic "lack of knowledge" does not only concern the patient's conscious awareness of her current state. Also, calling the process in question "repression" would require more attention to the patient's speech. At another moment, the same patient declares: "I am not very ambidextrous." In a Freudian reading (Freud, 1925), the sentence could be considered as a *negation*, i.e., a process which permits a partial lifting of repression. The negative form allows the subject to express what poses a question to him, yet without agreeing with what he is saying. In this way, we could hear the patient saying, without admitting it, "I *am* very ambidextrous". Her words might also be considered as an understatement or euphemism, meaning "I am bad at using both hands", or "I am only good at using one hand". What all these formulations have in common is leaving aside either the unilateral deficiency or its recent onset.

Kaplan-Solms and Solms (2000) also provide a psychoanalytic interpretation in terms of repression. According to them, the patient represses the negative emotions stirred by his disability, while these emotions are expressed when the patient is confronted with fictional narrative or external events that evoke disability, or if the psychoanalyst confronts the patient with his difficulties. Still, we should remember that the expression of such emotions may be quite compatible with the patient's manifest ignorance of hemiplegia: We often see patients who complain bitterly of having lost their independence, having become "a vegetable" or having to use a wheelchair, but never mention the motor deficiency responsible for their misfortune (see for example, Morin, Thibierge and Perrigot, 2001).

Anosognosia: the result of a regression to primary narcissism?

Kaplan-Solms and Solms (2000) also provide a second psychoanalytic interpretation. Because right-hemisphere lesions are known to affect spatial representation, they might also abolish the distance which separates the subject from the object. This would imply a regression to the state of primary narcissism, a state in which the subject does not conceive of any separation between his own body and the objects that bring him pleasure and satisfaction. In this theory, the paralysed limbs would no longer be invested by the libido and, as a result, would be perceived as a hated part of reality. This would account for both anosognosia and the xenopathic tone of somatoparaphrenia. This theory raises many questions. The relationship between psychic space and geometric space is only based on a verbal analogy. But more importantly, the authors' latter hypothesis (anosognosia is due to a regression to primary narcissism) contradicts the former (anosognosia is due to repression). If the patient has indeed regressed to primary narcissism and thus cannot recognise certain objects as external to himself, how do we conceive of his capacity for self-representation? In other words, from what point of view could he think of his paralysis as unbearable and repress his negative emotions? Nevertheless, the latter hypothesis arrives at the very conclusion we have reached as well, by another path; i.e., in RHS patients the paralysed limbs can assume an object-like status. However, in our hypothesis, this would result from a *lifting* of primary repression, rather that an excess of neurotic (secondary) repression.

Anosognosia: a structural reading

Trying to understand anosognosia, we must meet several methodological conditions. First, we must establish how anosognosia differs from the psychological reactions of recently disabled non-RHS patients, hemiplegic or not, with or without a brain injury. Second, we must examine the relationships of anosognosia with body schema disorders. To do so, patients must be interviewed in a way that avoids suggestion. We must be careful not to apply any kind of psychological interpretation before studying the patients' discourse. In the next section, we will follow these rules to examine some of the data and observations reported earlier.

Anosognosia in left hemiplegia is not a neurotic méconnaissance

Whether hemiplegic or not, most of the patients who have recently suffered a disability (Morin and Salazar-Orvig, 1996) share certain characteristics. As I have discussed previously, when such patients are speaking of themselves, they use grammatical subjects in a particular way. Let us take a typical sentence: "What bothers me most is that one is dependent on one's relatives" [*Je suis surtout gênée parce qu'on est tributaire de tous les siens*]. This formulation shows that the patient maintains a point of view on what she is experiencing (*It bothers me*, literally, *I am bothered* ["Je suis gênée"]), but hesitates to take on the image of what she has become ("one is dependent" [*on est tributaire*]). Hemiplegic patients describe their deficiencies with physiologically adequate terms ("I cannot control my hand, I cannot feel when I am touched" [*Je ne peux pas commander ma main, je ne sens pas quand on me touche*]). And yet, surprisingly, their self-portraits do not show the concrete aspects of their disability. All portraits look symmetrical, whether the patient presents with a symmetrical deficiency (paraplegia) or not (unilateral fracture or hemiplegia). Non-RHS patients, who do not present with anosognosia, are able to describe their deficiencies but seem not to fully accept their altered image. Such an attitude belongs to the normal neurotic *méconnaissance*, a stage that allows us to experience and overcome different kinds of loss and mourning.

Anosognosia in left hemiplegia is associated with body image disorders

The discourse and self-portraits of RHS patients are quite different. A highly typical trait of discourse is the expression "they say that . . ." [*on dit que . . .*] – that I am making progress, that I do or don't try hard enough, that I have hemiplegia etc. – the pronoun "they" referring to doctors, physiotherapists and other people involved. The patient thus does not seem to be personally involved not only in his illness or deficiency, but even in the assessment of his recovery. It is as if these patients lacked self-representation, an image of oneself that would provide them with a stable point of view to consider their current condition. RHS patients might describe the appearance of their paralysed limb (its colour or texture), rather than their deficiency; there is a significant correlation between this trait and the presence of hemineglect (Morin, Timsit et al., 2003). They personify their paralysed arm or hand: "I have a rubber hand which does not answer my calls"; "the arm is like myself, it has worked too much and would like to stop" (Morin, Durand et al., 2003). Their self-portraits may be altered by hemineglect, but they are also disorganised and fragmented, and the patients neither notice nor correct these anomalies (Morin, Pradat-Diehl, Robain, Bensalah and Perrigot, 2003). They often draw their wheelchair, cane or sling (see Figures 5.1, 5.4, 6.1 and 6.8). All these characteristics contrast with those of the portraits drawn by non-RHS patients: The body image is fragmented and patients not only comment on the appearance of their limbs, but also include the stigmatising equipment related to the disability.

Unlike neurotic *méconnaissance*, anosognosia in left hemiplegia does not resemble a psychological phenomenon we could understand intuitively, by identifying with a hemiplegic patient.[2] Therefore, in order to understand it better, we must look at the different psychic symptoms of RHS, in particular somatoparaphrenia (Gertsmann, 1942). Patients presenting with somatoparaphrenia speak of their paralysed hand as if it were another person or belonged to another person. Although somatoparaphrenia is considered rare (Baier and Karnath, 2008), its milder forms can be found in many RHS patients (Morin, Timsit et al., 2003). In somatoparaphrenia, the subject no longer considers himself as a whole and coherent being. In psychoanalytic terms, we could say that his body image is fragmented.

Anosognosia, body image and the object

We have shown that in patients with somatoparaphrenia (Morin, Thibierge, Bruguière, Pradat-Diehl and Mazevet, 2005), asomatognosia (Morin, Durand et al., 2003) or hemineglect (Morin, Thibierge and Perrigot, 2001) the disorganization of body schema and body image can go hand in hand with pathological manifestations of the object, in the psychoanalytic sense of the term. The self-portraits drawn by Mr E (Morin, Thibierge and Perrigot, 2001) were either "completely messed up", "monkey-like" or figures with the left-hand limbs missing (see Figures 6.1, 6.2 and 6.3). The fragmentation of body image was therefore associated with the representation of a dehumanised being. When talking of their paralysed arm, two asomatognosic patients spoke about kissing and biting (Morin, Durand et al., 2003). In several female patients (Morin, Thibierge, Bruguière et al., 2005) the disorganisation of body image coexisted with the appearance of a fictitious or real daughter replacing the hemiplegic hand. These cases led us to argue that anosognosia might be related to the object's sudden intrusion into the patient's psychic life (Morin and Thibierge, 2004).

We must remember that from the psychoanalytic point of view a normal cognitive functioning means being able to orient oneself in a recognisable, familiar reality, to 'function' without the need to think of or to be affected by everything we do. This implies that the object is neutralised, not identified (Thibierge, 2011). The object's 'revelation' can therefore block the patient's view on things, preventing him from acknowledging reality, including the bodily reality of hemiplegia. This might account for the fact that the anosognosic patient does not question the validity of his perception or try to distance himself from his symptoms. It might also explain the variability of anosognosia, the fact that some elements of reality might be perceived but not others.

More generally, based on the relationships between image and the object, we could put forth an interpretation of the cognitive disorders of RHS. In its neutralised, repressed or metaphorical form, the lost object animates our psychic life, even when we are engaged in completely routine activities, those we perform 'on autopilot'. Yet, for example, Mr E's drawing of himself as a trout fisher (Figure 6.2) suggests that after an RBI this might no longer be possible. It is only through this reminder of his youthful manliness that the patient can overcome his left hemineglect and draw a phallic symbol. Following this line of thinking, we could argue that in RHS, the actual presence of the object, rather than its neutralised form, becomes necessary to sustain, albeit only momentarily, what we would consider normal cognitive activity.

Notes

1 In French psychoanalysis, *déni* as the equivalent of "denial" evokes the Freudian *Verleugnung* rather than the neurotic repression.
2 This is indeed the way Weinstein and Kahn reasoned in their book *Denial of Illness* (1955).

References

Adair, J.C., Barrett, A.M. (2011). Anosognosia. In K.M. Heilman and E. Valenstein (Eds.), *Cognitive Neuropsychology* (pp. 198–214). New York: Oxford University Press.

Babinski, J. (1914). Contribution à l'étude des troubles mentaux dans l'hémiplégie organique cérébrale (anosognosie). *Revue Neurologique (Paris)*, *1*, 845–848.

Baier, B., Karnath, H.O. (2008). Tight link between our sense of limb ownership and self-awareness of actions. *Stroke*, *39*, 486–488.

Borel, J. (1931). *Les méconnaissances systématiques chez l'aliéné. La méconnaissance de la mort*. Medical thesis. Paris: Arnette.

Cappa, S., Sterzi, R., Vallar, G., Bisiach, E. (1987). Remission of hemineglect and anosognosia during vestibular stimulation. *Neuropsychologia*, *25*, 775–782.

Czermak, M. (1998). On m'arlequine la mentalité. Du caractère irrésistible et traumatique du transfert dans les psychoses. J. Bergès (Ed.), *Patronymies. Considérations cliniques sur les psychoses* (pp. 96–101). Paris: Masson.

Delahousse, J. (1972). Considérations sur l'attitude anosognosique de l'hémiplégique gauche. In *Actes du 70ᵉ Congrès de Psychiatrie et de Neurologie* (pp. 1082–1088). Paris: Masson.

Dissez, N. (2009). Histoire d'un concept psychiatrique tombé dans l'oubli: la méconnaissance systématique, ou Lacan sur la trace de la forclusion du symbolique. *Revue Lacanienne*, *5*, 188–200.

Ellis, S.J., Small, M. (1993). Denial of illness in stroke. *Stroke*, *24*, 757–759.

Freud, S. (1925). Negation. *Standard Edition*, *19*, 235–239.

Freud, S. (1938). Splitting of the ego in the process of defence. *Standard Edition*, *23*, 271–272.

Gertsmann, J. (1942). Problems in imperception of disease and of impaired body with organic lesions. *Archives of Neurology and Psychiatry*, *48*, 890–913.

Geschwind, N. (1965). Disconnexion syndromes in animals and man. *Brain*, *88*, 237–294.

Kaplan-Solms, K., Solms, M. (2000). *Clinical Studies in Neuro-Psychoanalysis: Introduction to a Depth Neuropsychology.* London: Karnac Books.

Morin, C., Durand, E., Marchal, F., Timsit, S., Manai, R., Pradat-Diehl, P., Rancurel, G. (2003). Asomatognosie et troubles de l'oralité: Une lecture psychanalytique. *Annales de Réadaptation et de Médecine Physique*, *46*, 12–23.

Morin, C., Pradat-Diehl, P., Robain, G., Bensalah, Y., Perrigot, M. (2003). Stroke hemiplegia and specular image: Lessons from self-portraits. *International Journal of Human Aging and Development*, *56*, 1–41.

Morin, C., Salazar-Orvig, A. (1996). Paroles de patients hémiplégiques: discours et position subjective. *Sciences Sociales et Santé*, *14*, 47–78.

Morin, C., Thibierge, S. (2004). L'image du corps en neurologie: de la cénesthésie à l'image spéculaire. Apports cliniques et théoriques de la psychanalyse. *L'Evolution Psychiatrique*, *69*, 417–430.

Morin, C., Thibierge, S., Bruguière, P., Pradat-Diehl, P., Mazevet, D. (2005). "Daughter-somatoparaphrenia" in women with right hemisphere syndrome: A psychoanalytical perspective on neurological body knowledge disorders. *Neuropsychoanalysis*, *7*, 47–60.

Morin, C., Thibierge, S., Perrigot, M. (2001). Right brain damage, body image and language: A psychoanalytic perspective. *Journal of Mind and Behavior*, *22*, 69–89.

Morin, C., Timsit, S., Durand, E., Marchal, F., Manai, R., Perrigot, M., Pradat-Diehl, P., Rancurel, G. (2003). Discours sur la main, asomatognosie et héminégligence. *Annales de Réadaptation et de Médecine Physique*, *46*, 514.

Ramachandran, V.S., Blakeslee, S. (1998). *Phantoms in the Brain: Probing the Mysteries of the Human Mind.* New York: William Morrow.

Thibierge, S. (2011). *Le nom, l'image, l'objet. Image du corps et reconnaissance.* Paris: PUF.

Vocat, R. (2010). *L'anosognosie. Un siècle de recherches.* Sarrebrück: Editions Universitaires Européennes.

Weinstein, E.A., Kahn, R.L. (1955). *Denial of Illness.* Springfield: C.C. Thomas.

Chapter 9

Right-hemisphere syndrome and pathological mourning

Neurological literature is rich with studies devoted to the emotional disorders and depression that may result from a stroke. According to Robinson (2006), depression is more often observed after left anterior brain lesions, while mania typically occurs after right brain lesions. Bogousslavsky (2003) considers that sadness is less frequently seen in right hemispheric lesions than in left lesions but that in right lesions sadness and indifference are related to anosognosia. However, comparatively little has been written about the patients' process of mourning. In fact, we cannot equate depressive mood with the mourning process, even though every mourning subject is expected to go through a depressive phase before coping with his new situation. It seems more adequate to underline that in any mourning process the subject must withdraw libido from his body image, the slow and detailed work Freud described in *Mourning and Melancholia* (1917). This is apparent in a study looking at the recovery process of eight patients enrolled in a "stroke recovery school" (Roman, 2008). Patients may attend the school activities for several years. They are offered rehabilitation sessions and also collectively participate in everyday activities. For the author of the study, who conducted a series of interviews with each patient, the most striking psychological aspect of recovery is the anxiety caused by what she calls the "psycho-traumatic aspects" of stroke. Interestingly, she notes that patients may be crying desperately when alone, but at other times insist that they have never lost hope; they may participate in school activities while carefully avoiding mirrors. The three-year period post stroke generally marks a turn in patients' narcissistic recovery, although even later they may very well continue to make significant cognitive progress. For example, it is around this time that a patient declares that "she's beginning to like the person she is now."

These observations, which align with our own clinical experience, correspond to various aspects of a normal process of mourning. It is noteworthy that all the eight patients described in the study presented with left brain lesions; in other words, none of the patients who volunteered to participate in a long-term process of rehabilitation and conversations with their therapists, who accepted to face mourning and rehabilitation simultaneously, presented with RBI. This may seem surprising, since, due to language problems, patients with left brain injury are generally not recruited to take part in studies which involve interviews and dialogues. This might indirectly suggest that RBI patients did not volunteer or did not persist in attending the school's activities and that their way of undergoing the mourning process differs from other patients.

Indeed, we cannot expect a normal mourning process to be compatible with pathological narcissism. Kaplan-Solms and Solms (2000) discussed five cases of RBI patients having psychoanalytic therapy (several sessions weekly) during the first months after their stroke. They characterise the psychical symptomatology of these patients as a variety of narcissistic disorders: narcissistic withdrawal, "brittle narcissism", melancholic or paranoiac reactions. Based on their observations, the authors make a rather bold suggestion that the right hemisphere is the "neuropsychological vehicle" of the normal object cathexis. In their understanding, such normal investment would consist in loving the object and recognising it as a whole object, clearly separated from the subject. Insofar as they disturb the subject's spatial representation, right hemispheric lesions would abolish the gap between the subject and the object. As a result, the subject would regress to primary narcissism, a state in which no separation is made between his body and the objects that provide pleasure and satisfaction, and all sources of unpleasure are expelled outwards. Thereafter, the paralysed limbs, which are outside the patient's control, would lose their libidinal cathexis and be seen as a hated part of the external world. This would prevent the patients from being able to mourn the command of their hand (or more generally to mourn their past life). Although this interpretation, which Solms also applies to anosognosia (Kaplan-Solms and Solms, 2000), relies on an understanding of the subject-object relationship that is quite different from our own conception above, it is interesting to note that both theories analyse RBI cases and interpret them in terms of a disorder of the subject-object relationship.

Clinically, the recovery process of RBI patients with body image disorders clearly differs from the mourning observed in both healthy subjects and in hemiplegic patients devoid of body image disorders. The case of Mrs N, who was "consoled" by the presence of her embodied daughter-hand and never became depressed, is exemplary. Such behaviour is fundamentally different from the ordinary mourning process, where on the contrary the subject is inconsolable. A formula put forward by Abraham and Torok (1972) seems to sum up this difference very well. According to them, mourning normally consists of an *introjection*, which the authors understand as "fantasizing swallowing what is lost". They write: "In order not to have to 'swallow' a loss, we fantasize swallowing (or having swallowed) that which has been lost as if it were some kind of thing" (1972, p. 68). This formulation illustrates the antinomy of mourning (losing) versus retaining the object. In the daughter-hand cases we have described above, the object is embodied, not introjected; the loss is not symbolised; in other words, no mourning has taken place. However, we must specify that our systematic observations only concern patients seen within the first months after their stroke. My clinical experience suggests that RHS patients may retain the same attitude towards their disability over the long term and that this is very different from the recovery of other patients. Two opposing clinical examples will illustrate this difference.

Mr R, whose initial symptoms have been described in Chapter 6, attended therapy in the rehabilitation department for several years. He continued to present with a complete paralysis of both his hand and his arm; he never returned to his managerial position and instead devoted his time to a variety of hobbies (filing his photography and stamp collections, travelling and visiting expositions). Mr R was well aware that he had attention and memory disorders: reading and writing took great effort and he had a "hard time producing anything logical in writing". After three years, Mr R declared that he enjoyed his life and "would not think of complaining"; he had "found a little oasis" and was again interested in going out. Despite many complications (such as falls and epileptic seizures), Mr R said: "One tries to make the old fellow function as well as possible" [*On essaye de faire marcher le bonhomme le mieux possible*]. Things were perhaps not so simple: His wife told me she would "use any chance she had to go away" because she felt burnt out. The patient never stopped either his cognitive rehabilitation or his physical therapy – he was convinced that without the latter, he could not go outside. In reality, Mr R seemed obsessed by an anxious concern about keeping his left shoulder "in place". He spoke of this worry during several sessions, because he had problems finding and keeping physiotherapists able to manage this operation. More surprisingly, once I was talking with Mr R about the potential benefits of losing a little weight when he explained to me that "he could make his bowels function" only "when his body had a certain shape", which could not be guaranteed below a hundred kilos. During the first year after his discharge from hospital, Mr R repeatedly commented on some modest progress he had observed in the use of his left hand. He always used the same words: "I eat slices of sausage with my left hand." What he meant is that he used his left hand to hold the sausage while slicing it, and then, with much difficulty, to put the slices into his mouth. During the later course of his rehabilitation, Mr R remained very concerned about keeping his shoulder in a painless position. In his opinion, the pain derived from the serratus anterior muscle (but as he often forgot the name his physiotherapist gave to this muscle, Mr. R preferred to call it "the great pain in the neck" [*le grand emmerdeur*]). The pain then descended "until it reached the quadriceps", i.e., anatomically speaking, it followed no logical path. In a self-portrait Mr R drew five years after his stroke (Figure 9.1), the left shoulder is indeed not in the correct position, because both arms are directly attached to the neck. The representation of hands is asymmetrical. Hemineglect is modest – the left ear is missing, and one eye is drawn with a heavier line, a black eye, as Mr R commented afterwards. The left arm and leg seem to drag the entire Figure downwards. The picture reveals a disorder of specular image: Mr R's arm remains in the position of the oral object (remember that at the very beginning of his illness, Mr R felt like biting a left arm); the rehabilitation will go on indefinitely, the left shoulder will never be correctly positioned, the body image has lost its axis. The question then arises: What kind of mourning did Mr R undergo to manifestly accept living with his sequelae while still being troubled by a shoulder that can never be put in the correct position?

The picture is quite different in patients who have no body schema disorders. Mr C's case is very illustrative. This patient suffered a right hemiplegia and severe aphasia due to a left brain CVA. When I met him two years after his stroke, his therapists had become worried because he kept repeating: "Death! Death!" From then on we met once a week.

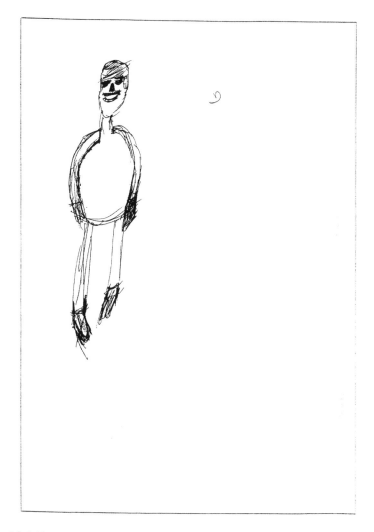

Figure 9.1 Self-portrait of a right-handed patient with body schema disorders, Mr R, three years after his CVA
One ear is lacking on the left due to hemineglect. The patient blackens the eye on the left and says he has drawn a black eye.

Using drawings and writing, Mr C told me what was worrying him. His stroke had happened in a context of great anxiety, at a time when he was fearing for his son's life. Mr C felt a need to speak about this trauma. He complained bitterly about his disordered language. In our first meetings,

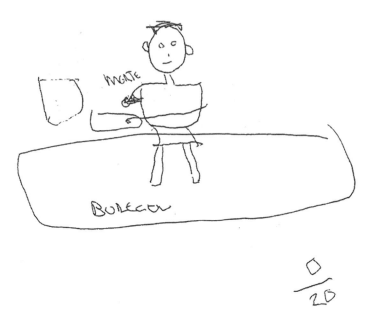

Figure 9.2 Self-portrait of a right-handed patient without body schema disorders (left CVA), six years after his stroke
Mr C working at his desk ["*bureau*"] in front of his computer. He wrote the word "*morte*" [dead] above his paralysed arm.

he would often write a single word: "Speech!" Mr C attended regular speech therapy sessions as an outpatient for several years, eventually recovering a non-grammatical but understandable speech. He returned to the company which had employed him before, but was aware that his new job there was neither greatly productive nor valuable. He travelled, visited his sons and grandchildren, managed his financial affairs and estate properties. Eventually he stopped all rehabilitation activities. Mr C never spontaneously spoke of his paralysed arm, the use of which he had lost completely. A self-portrait made six years after his stroke presents him sitting at his desk before his computer (Figure 9.2). The right hand, "dead", as Mr C writes, is darkened and looks atrophic. Mr C writes "0/20", not without smiling. It is unclear if the zero rates his drawing or himself. We do not know either if Mr C has now "accepted his disability" in line with the supposedly normal mourning process. However, we can see that, while being perfectly aware of what his difficulties consist in, he no longer devotes his entire life to treating them.

References

Abraham, N., Torok, M. (1972). Introjecter-incorporer: deuil ou mélancolie. *Nouvelle Revue de Psychanalyse, 6,* 111–122.

Bogousslavsky, J. (2003). William Feinberg lecture 2002: Emotions, mood, and behavior after stroke. *Stroke, 34,* 1046–1050.

Freud, S. (1917). Mourning and melancholia. *Standard Edition, 14,* 245–258.

Kaplan-Solms, K., Solms, M. (2000). *Clinical Studies in Neuro-Psychoanalysis: Introduction to a Depth Neuropsychology.* London: Karnac Books.

Robinson, R.G. (2006). *The Clinical Neuropsychiatry of Stroke: Cognitive, Behavioral Emotional Disorders Following Vascular Brain Injury.* Cambridge: Cambridge University Press.

Roman, M.W. (2008). Lessons learned from a school for stroke recovery. *Topics in Stroke Rehabilitation, 15,* 59–71.

Conclusion

Having come to the end of this theoretical and clinical journey, it is time to ask: What did we learn?

We have put the psychoanalytic concept of the object-image relationship to the test, by comparing disabled patients with and without body image and body schema disorders. The words and drawings of patients with body image disorders have corroborated our hypothesis that a stable body image cannot be maintained unless the object is repressed. In some RHS patients (as is the case in everyday psychopathology, in both neurosis and psychosis) the fragmentation of body image goes hand in hand with the lifting of repression of the object. We have also shown how certain signifiers of the object are attached to specific parts of our bodies, thus bringing our bodies into the discourse that supports our lives.

What do these conclusions mean for the clinical practice of neurology and post-stroke rehabilitation? First, our observations invite us to take a step back from our medical training, which can easily lead us to "neurologise" every symptom and interpret it in terms of a cognitive dysfunction. Still, we should remain equally sceptical of all attempts at "psychologising" it. These tendencies are in fact two sides of the same coin and we encounter them as soon as we start wondering about the "psychological functioning" of these patients, as if their brain injury had transformed them into a species quite different from ourselves and open to our observation. And yet, the basic elements of our psychic structure, whether they are knotted together harmoniously or simply loosely attached, are common to all speaking beings. Giving his book the title *L'image de* notre *corps* [The image of *our* body], this premise seems to have been very much on Lhermitte's mind.

This is not to deny that a brain injury can produce a change or indeed a deficit in cerebral functioning. This of course must be taken into account and being able to do so is simply part of our job. As neurologists or rehabilitation therapists, doing our job well means observing and listening to the patients, in order to bring their neurological symptoms to light. I am using the word *listening* on purpose, despite its often being loaded with various psychologising notions. That in order to assess a patient's subjective position vis-à-vis his illness we must first listen to him is simply obvious. However, carefully listening to the patient's words is also the best way to understand the actual nature of his pathology, as our study of body image disorders plainly shows.

Thanks to this type of listening, we have been able to use the speech and self-portraits of stroke patients to learn to distinguish between two types of hemiplegic patients: (1) those who suffer from only a disorder of body perception or command (what we could call *simple hemiplegia*) and (2) those who also present with a body image disorder (*complicated hemiplegia*). The question then arises: What are the implications of this distinction for patient care? In cases of simple hemiplegia, there is a general assumption that we know how to deal with patients whose behaviour and discourse do not appear strange to us. However, such confidence is rather paradoxical. In fact, by identifying with the narcissistically injured patients, we gain little insight into what their image conceals, namely the object which animates the patient's desire to recover and live a full life, and of which we ordinarily know nothing. Patients' trust in their therapists, i.e., the transferential relationship that is formed between them, is one of the factors that help patients get better, but *how* this happens usually remains outside our perception.

As for patients with body image alterations, the data presented in this book might be a starting point for looking at new methods of rehabilitation. All therapists know that RHS may present a serious challenge to their efforts, insofar as the body image disorder undermines the basis for both the 'motivation' and the 'awareness' that are supposed to be essential prerequisites for any process of rehabilitation. Fotopoulou, Rudd, Holmes and Kopelman (2009) have observed patients whose anosognosia was alleviated after watching a video of their own performance. We are currently looking at various aspects of the relationship RHS patients have to their mirror image. However, we should be rather prudent, because one of the lessons of our research presented in this book is the ability of organic brain lesions to alter body image. Because body image determines our perceptions (and, we might add, our thoughts), its alteration proves resistant to "orthopaedic" re-education, to various attempts at "resuscitating the body schema", to pedagogical explanations and psychological interpretations (Kortte and Hillis, 2011). Most often we must simply learn to follow the patient's own journey and patiently wait for a spontaneous recovery, the mechanisms of which are still largely unclear. "Simply" is perhaps not the right term. In fact, is it really so simple to offer our patience to persons with an altered body image, who could otherwise see – and often do see – our insistence on correcting and improving their posture, movement and attention as aggressive, infantilising or disrespectful?

Lastly, the disentangling of the link between the image and object in somatoparaphrenia can teach us a great deal about the coordinates of the object in a given patient, perhaps more than what the patient knows about it himself. But paradoxically, this knowledge, to which the patient seems to have no access, is of no therapeutic use. Knowing does not increase our therapeutic power.

References

Fotopoulou, A., Rudd, A., Holmes, P., Kopelman, M. (2009). Self-observation reinstates motor awareness in anosognosia for hemiplegia. *Neuropsychologia*, *47*, 1256–1260.

Kortte, K.B., Hillis, A.E. (2011). Recent trends in rehabilitation interventions for visual neglect and anosognosia for hemiplegia following right hemisphere stroke. *Future Neurology*, *6*, 33–43.

Index